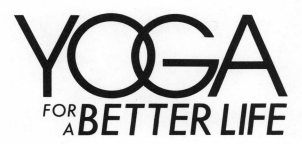

Cover art by Jane A. Evans
Photographs by J. Ramanan

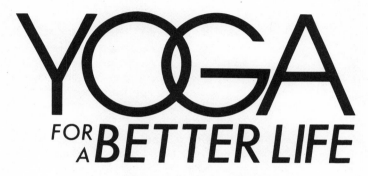

YOGA
FOR A BETTER LIFE

HOW TO COMPOSE
YOUR OWN COMPLETE YOGA COURSE

by *DAVID SCHONFELD*

QUEST BOOKS

*This publication made possible with
the assistance of the Kern Foundation.*

**The Theosophical Publishing House
Wheaton, IL/Madras, India/London, England**

Quest Books are published by The Theosophical
Publishing House, a department of The Theosophical
Society in America.

Library of Congress Cataloging in Publication Data

Schonfeld, David, 1946-
        Yoga for a better life.

        (A Quest book)
        1. Yoga, Hatha. I. Title.
        RA781.7.S3   613.7'046   79-6548
        ISBN 0-8356-0536-1 (pbk.)

Printed in the United States of America

CONTENTS

Introduction 1

Chapter 1
Sound Mind, Sound Body 5

Chapter 2
Questions and Answers 16

Chapter 3
A Model Practice Sequence 24

Chapter 4
Explaining the Sequence 31

Chapter 5
An Anthology of Asanas 44

Chapter 6
Yoga and the Breath 74

Chapter 7
Headstand: How and Why 84

Chapter 8
Elements of Pranayama 98

Chapter 9
Composing Your Own Course 111

References and Notes 125

ACKNOWLEDGEMENTS

We acknowledge our gratitude to the following publishers for permission to reprint their works of authorship:

Excerpted from the book, *Breakfast of Champions* by Kurt Vonnegut, Jr. Copyright © 1973 by Kurt Vonnegut, Jr. Reprinted by permission of Delacorte Press/Seymour Lawrence.

Excerpts from *Plagues and Peoples* by William H. McNeill. Copyright © 1976 by William H. McNeill. Reprinted by permission of Doubleday & Co., Inc.

Dr. F. Chandra, *The Medical and Physiological Aspects of Headstand* (Somerset, England: Cambridge Yoga Publications).

T.K.V. Desikachar, *Religiousness in Yoga: Lectures on Theory and Practice.* Edited by Mary Louise Skelton and John Ross Carter (Washington, D.C.: University Press of America, 1980).

Taken from *Yoga and Medicine* by Steven F. Brena, M.D., © 1972. Used by permission of Julian Press.

Excerpts from *The Invincible Pyramid* by Loren Eisely, and *The Shape of Intelligence* by H. Chandler Elliott, by permission of Charles Scribner's Sons.

Special gratitude to:

Mr. J. Ramanan, a young man of many talents who did the photography so eagerly and expertly.

Mr. K. Padmanabhan, ever obliging; and to Nicole Nordby-Marcault, Sheila Richards, and Bill Buckland (fellow students at the Krishnamacharya Yoga Mandiram) who so cooperatively volunteered to be photographed.

Didi, whose generous hospitality allowed me to revise the manuscript in the pleasant surrounding of Kathmandu.

The many friends who encouraged me and offered suggestions.

My family, for its loving support throughout my long sojourns in India.

Amy Ruth Catlin, without whom I could not have returned to Madras so soon.

To my teacher, Sri T.K.V. Desikachar, I owe an immense debt of gratitude. It was he who introduced me to Yoga and suggested I write this book. Without his guidance throughout, it would never have materialized.

I am fortunate to have had a long association with Desikachar, and I have tried to convey something of the spirit of his teaching. But I am not his designated mouthpiece, nor is this his book. For its errors and lapses I alone am responsible.

INTRODUCTION

This book is about Yoga and *your* life, but you may well ask what it has done for mine.

Why did I first turn to Yoga? It was May 1972, and as I recall it now I was restless, unhappy, and at odds with myself. I had gone to India to study music, but as the hot season came on I became too incapacitated to have energy for anything but sleeping.

I had been living for months near a world-renowned Yoga school, and had met many persons who had come from afar to undergo training there. I was curious about what they were doing, but quite skeptical. I wasn't attracted by what I took to be the religious connotations of Yoga and knew nothing of its philosophical basis. It was only when I began to feel desperate and nothing seemed to help that I resolved to give Yoga a try.

In response to my inquiry, T.K.V. Desikachar agreed to take me as a private student. He asked me to come once a week for a 45-minute lesson and explained that I must practice every day the material he gave me during the lesson. The exercises he gave me were so pleasurable that I needed no prodding. On the contrary, Desikachar cautioned me not to overdo it. He told me to practice only once a day, not for too long, ideally in the late afternoon when my body was least stiff. As I became more adept he let me decide for myself what, when, and for how long to practice.

My teacher's manner right away put me at ease. He never prescribed any code of conduct or dietary restrictions. In fact, he listened good-naturedly when I tried to persuade *him* to sample the excellent fresh fish available in Madras! We followed no ritual; there were no Hindu prayers or Sanskrit mantras. Instead of the ancient, austere guru I was expecting, Desikachar turned out to be young, attractive, unassuming, and friendly.

An honors graduate, he had been a successful civil engineer before gradually switching over to full-time Yoga teaching. Though earning less money, he has had the satisfaction of sharing with others what he received from his father and teacher, Sri T. Krishnamacharya—himself an eminent Yoga master and scion of a long tradition.

My lessons were held in a studio in the family home. Desikachar has always been reluctant to establish any kind of "ashram." He does not wish to be omnipresent, to impose disciplines on people or limit their freedom. He tries to keep a low profile and spends what free time he has with his family. Like all his students, I would have liked more time with him. But I couldn't complain. In one private lesson I got more than enough to motivate me and keep me seriously practicing until the next week. When we began to consider questions of therapy and pedagogy he increased my lessons to two and then three a week.

1

I was never conscious of a syllabus, or of a deadline for mastering a given posture. My teacher was giving me what he thought I needed, at just the pace at which I was able to progress. If sometimes I felt he was pushing me, it was no doubt because he wanted to prove to me that I was capable of more than I realized. Had I been overeager or reckless he would have restrained me.

If I showed up with a cold or a headache or a stomachache or a lack of sleep, he would give me a milder, less orthodox course. I found it disconcerting at first that, when I would come in feeling miserable, Desikachar's face would brighten. What excited him was not my suffering, of course, but the prospect of alleviating it swiftly through Yoga.

Very quickly my idiosyncrasies emerged. Whether from my playing a musical instrument or having driven a taxi for a year, my neck and shoulders, I discovered, were extremely stiff. I could turn my head one way but not the other. My displeasure at having this problem brought to my attention was soon outweighed by my joy in seeing the problem disappear. Before Yoga I could only sleep on my belly, with my head turned to one side. Within a month or two I was falling asleep on my back, without a pillow even, and would awake refreshed, with no tension in my neck muscles.

Likewise, I learned that one hip was stiffer than the other, and practiced exercises to equalize them. In time, deeper problems surfaced and gradually diminished: a stiff back, stiff legs, weak wrists, under-developed back muscles, eyestrain. Attempting balancing exercises, I came to grips with deep-seated fears of losing control. The thought of standing on my head once terrified me; my first headstand without wall support—after seven months of lessons—was a triumph.

To my great delight I *did* become less restless, happier, and less at odds with myself. Moreover, I felt I had started to grow younger instead of older. For once I seemed to be *leading* my life instead of being led.

My posture became straight and effortless. I felt my lung capacity increase, and began to enjoy breathing as never before. Tastes and fragrances took on new subtlety as my sinuses cleared up. I was more relaxed and energetic during the day, and slept more soundly at night. Hot weather no longer incapacitated me. My digestion improved. My abdominal muscles firmed up and I lost excess weight. I became less impetuous and less clumsy, no longer inflicting frequent cuts and bruises on myself. Not only could I sit still for long periods, but I could do so in cross-legged positions which, prior to Yoga, had been excruciating. That alone was worth it to me, since physical discomfort had greatly impeded my music practice. (The South Indian vīnā must be played seated cross-legged on the floor.)

To be sure, even with Yoga my life was not without difficulties. During one period I was under great emotional stress because of a deteriorating relationship. I might have used all my time with my teacher unburdening myself, but he preferred instead to give me physical exercises. These were surprisingly helpful in relaxing tension and calming my mind. My situation always looked less bleak after those sessions. Equally as effective as the exercise therapy Desikachar was giving me was the advice he gave me every week, his arm draped across my shoulders. "Take life easy, sir," he would tell me.

When, after some time, I began inquiring about the philosophy underlying Yoga practice, Desikachar proposed a study of the *Yoga Sutra*. He taught the verses to my two classmates and me in the traditional way, interpreted their meaning, and encouraged us to relate them to our own experiences and observations. We went very slowly, often spending several hours on a single pregnant phrase. Yet nine months of such encounters did not dull our enthusiasm.

In the same patient and painstaking spirit, Desikachar helped me to see this book through to completion. Writing it required me to look more closely at my Yoga practice and the understanding behind it. I hope that you, the reader, will find this book a useful guide in your own explorations.

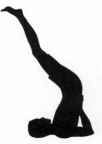

NOTE ON SANSKRIT

In transliterating Sanskrit words I have basically followed current scholarly practice; however, I have made a few substitutions, to help the general reader come closer to the correct pronunciation of certain consonants (e.g., *ch* for *c*, *sh* for *ś*, *sh* for *ṣ*, and *w* for *v* in some cases).

Approximate Value of the Vowels

a	as in m<u>o</u>ther
ā	as in f<u>a</u>ther
i	as in s<u>i</u>t
ī	as in s<u>ee</u>d
u	as in c<u>oo</u>k
ū	as in c<u>oo</u>l
ṛ	as in pe<u>r</u>suade (or p<u>r</u>etty)
ai	as in wh<u>i</u>te
e	as in f<u>a</u>ce
au	as in n<u>ow</u>
o	as in g<u>o</u>

Approximate Value of Problematic Consonants

1. Retroflex consonants: *ṭ, ḍ, ṇ, ṣh.*

    These are articulated like their equivalents in English, but with the tongue curled upward.

2. Dentals: *t, d.*

    These are not characteristic of English, but may be approximated by saying "<u>t</u>inker" with the tongue touching the teeth as for "<u>th</u>inker," or "<u>d</u>oze" with the tongue positioned for "<u>th</u>ose."

3. Aspirated stops: *kh, gh, ṭh, th, dh, ph, bh.*

    These are single consonants, like their unaspirated equivalents, but projected with a puff of air. Aspiration exists in English, but we are usually unconscious of it. The *p* in "punch," for example, would be heard as *ph* by an Indian.

    You can pronounce Sanskrit:

kh	as in wor<u>kh</u>orse
gh	as in do<u>gh</u>ouse
ṭh	as in ho<u>th</u>ouse
bh	as in clu<u>bh</u>ouse

1

SOUND MIND, SOUND BODY

Picture a people:
—living in uneasy peace;
—dependent on scarce resources and land pushed to maximum productivity;
—ethnically diverse and densely populated:
—urbanized, educated, and sophisticated;
—renowned for its arts and sciences;
—prosperous enough to be able to disdain materialism;
—leisured enough to question its work ethic;
—abounding in rival religions and cults;
—anxious about the future.

A description of contemporary Western civilization? Yes, but not exclusively. Earlier civilizations, in the course of their evolution, may have passed through a phase similar to the one we now are experiencing.

After man had exercised his talents in the building of the first neolithic cities and empires, a period mostly marked by architectural and military triumphs, an intellectual transformation descended upon the known world, a time of questioning. This era is fundamental to an understanding of man.... The period culminates in the first millennium before Christ. Here in the great centers of civilization, whether Chinese, Indian, Judaic, or Greek, man had begun to abandon inherited gods and purely tribal loyalties in favor of an inner world in which the pursuit of earthly power was ignored. The destiny of the human soul became of more significance than the looting of a province.... [This period] created the world of universal thought that is our most precious human heritage.[1]

We may trace our roots directly to Europe and the Mediterranean, but we should not overlook the influence Asia has had and still may have on us.

WHY INDIA?

Western skepticism about learning anything from India is understandable. India has been supine for centuries. But it was not always so. Once its civilization was as vigorous and vibrant as ours is today. Its reputation in the arts, sciences, and philosophy was worldwide.

Indian civilization, as we know it, was the result of a fusion between an earlier, indigenous culture and one brought from the northwest. Since then India has remained in contact with the West, mostly on the receiving end. Culturally and politically, India's sphere of influence extended in the opposite direction, toward Southeast Asia. Indian thought transformed the Orient.

5

Yet even in its heyday, Indian civilization remained fragile. One reason why, according to a recent provocative study by historian William H. McNeill, [2] has to do with the relation between the Indian climate and the prevalence of disease. On the plus side, India had fertile lands, cosmopolitan cities, a thriving foreign trade, and an abundant population. But the warm, humid Ganges flood plain was also an ideal environment for a wide variety of disease factors. McNeill speculates that even in relatively prosperous times the Indian peasantry suffered so much from debilitating illness that it could not provide the kind of food surplus necessary to fuel an imperial bureaucracy and its armies. India's material wealth may have been more fabled than real.

Weakened by disease, India was always vulnerable to attack—and attacked it was, time and time again. The irony is that the attackers were themselves vulnerable to the diseases they encountered. (When the events of Indian history are seen in the long view, it is never clear who was conqueror and who was conquered.) If civilization in India lacked the glorious epoch we associate with other civilizations, at least it never disappeared, as so many others have, but has persisted down to our time. Favored and handicapped alike by climatic, geographic and political forces, India evolved an attitude to life in keeping with its delicate ecology.

McNeill finds it not surprising, therefore, that the great religions which arose in India addressed themselves to a population in close touch with the hard realities of suffering and death. In McNeill's words,

> ...the two great Indian religions of Buddhism and Hinduism were fundamentally apolitical. Both, at least in theory, rejected worldly pomp, wealth, and power as mere illusion, along with everything else perceptible to the senses....Indian teachers...turned their backs on politics and society—in a sense despairing of it—and enjoined upon their followers a penurious way of life, minimizing their material demands on the environment in order to invite a liberating mystic vision more effectually. [3]

Nowadays we may decry what we see as the fatalism, negativism, or renunciation of Eastern philosophy, but we are reluctantly beginning to realize that short-range philosophies which presuppose unlimited resources and condone the exploitation of the natural environment are no longer acceptable. Like ancient India we appear to be wealthy, but our wealth too may be illusory. We have in our time apparently mastered the threat of decimation by infectious disease, but we have substituted demographic threats of even greater potency: mass starvation, global pollution, nuclear holocaust. If mankind survives its present predicament it may find itself turning more and more to an ethic strikingly resembling the transcendentalism of ancient India. It is largely for this reason that Hinduism and Buddhism seem increasingly appealing.

Without having to become Hindus or Buddhists, we in the West can at least tone down the intolerance and aggressiveness latent in our Judeo-Christian heritage, and learn to live peaceably on our precarious planet. And if it is really true that Indian teachers "turned their backs on politics and society," that is no reason why we must do so. Given the structure of our institutions, it would be disastrous if conscientious persons abandoned the public arena to demagogues and politicians. Indian religion may set little store by worldly success, but it nowhere advises complicity with wrongdoing.

What disturbs us most in the Indian ethos is probably the idea of self-mortification. As the above excerpt indicates, it must indeed have been prevalent at times, and with good reason. When calamity was always lurking in one form or another it made sense to be prepared for it through self-discipline. Only the strong could survive, and only the simple suffer no loss. Nevertheless, it is likely that this element in the Indian tradition has been exaggerated, precisely because it seems foreign to modern sensibilities. In Western history too there have been times when mortification had its adherents and its audience.

A careful reading of Hindu texts suggests that inflicting harm and suffering on oneself was actually a perversion of asceticism: a confusion of ends with means. The capacity to withstand extremes of climate, or physical stress, or emotion was not supposed to be the *substance* of asceticism, but one of its *results*. Many texts warn against extremes in daily living (in food, sex, labor, sleep, etc.), and insist that the body be properly cared for.

With all our prodigious attainments and unprecedented dilemmas, India may yet have something to teach us. The magnitude of our crisis is certainly new, but its nature is not; India has been here before. Looking outward has brought us great material benefits, but it has also brought us to the brink of disaster. Looking inward frightens us—we know we harbor demons—but have we still a choice?

As a distillation of ancient wisdom coupled to a timeless practical technique, Yoga offers a means of creative introspection which may be more relevant to us than we realize.

YOGA AND THE YOGA SUTRA

We do not know when Yoga began. It seems already to have been in practice at the time the earliest Aryan scriptures, the Vedas, were composed (ca. 1500-800 B.C.). But it was during the period of the Upanishads (ca. 800-200 B.C.), as Indian thinkers sought to comprehend the meaning of creation and the purpose of life, that Yoga rose to prominence.

The word *yoga*, according to a leading Sanskrit scholar, "is a fluid one, used in a variety of senses, philosophical and other....The root from which it is derived meant originally to 'hitch up', as horses to a vehicle; then figuratively, to 'put (anything) to active, vigorous, and purposeful use'.... [Yoga] may mean simply 'method, means'; and it is so used in the epic"[5] —i.e., the *Mahābhārata* (composed within the time span 400 B.C.-A.D. 400), which includes the famous *Bhagavad Gītā*. For example, the Gita contrasts the "method" of knowledge (*jñāna-yoga*) with the "method" of action (*karma-yoga*).

But Yoga as a way of salvation per se has another meaning than "method." "This other meaning is 'exertion, disciplined activity', a regular, disciplined course of *action* leading to a definite end; namely, the end of emancipation."[6]

In the Bhagavad Gita, Yoga sometimes means "remaining in worldly life and doing one's duty, without selfish interest."[7] In other Sanskrit texts, however, Yoga is normally used in the sense of "disciplined activity," the activity specifically implied being *dhyāna* (sometimes translated as "meditation"). But Yoga has yet another connotation in the classic text by Patanjali, the *Yoga Sūtra*.

The date of the Yoga Sutra is uncertain. Indian tradition places it back in the Upanishadic period, but some Western scholars argue for the fourth or fifth century A.D. What is beyond question, regardless of when it achieved its final form, is that the Yoga Sutra represents a very old science. It is remarkable for its eloquence and conciseness, and its primacy is accepted by all schools of Yoga. Furthermore, the Yoga Sutra is included as one of the six *darshanas*, or basic philosophical systems, of modern Hinduism.

A *sūtra* is a maxim or aphorism connected sequentially to other sutras. The word also refers to the entire compilation. The Yoga Sutra is made up of 195 sutras, divided into four parts or books. Let us turn to this work, at this point in our inquiry.

The second sutra of Part I defines Yoga as *chitta-vṛtti nirodha*: a state of mind in which, for a moment at least, there is full attention and accurate observation. The movement toward chitta-vrtti nirodha is analyzed in the first three sutras of Part III (which deals with the results of Yoga practice). First the mind is drawn to some object. Then it becomes more and more involved with the object. (This stage is *dhyāna*, the word being used here in a more technical sense.) Ultimately the perceiving mind transcends self-consciousness and, in effect, *merges* with the object. This is *samādhi*, and the clarity that ensues is, for Patanjali, the subtle meaning of Yoga.

THE MOMENT OF TRUTH

Part I of the Yoga Sutra (subtitled "On Samadhi"), looks into the implications of chitta-vrtti nirodha. The term *chitta-vṛtti* means "activity (singular or plural) of the mind." Patanjali recognizes five types of activity: correct cognition (through first-hand experience, inference, and authoritative testimony), erroneous cognition, imagination, sleep, and memory. The five activities are not in themselves good or bad, but may have positive or negative consequences (I.5-11).

"Mind" in Yoga theory, does not include the entire territory of consciousness, as it generally does in Western usage. The functions we ascribe to "mind" are divided, in Yoga, between *chitta*—responsible for all thinking and feeling—and *puruṣa*, which is conceived of as pure consciousness: that which animates the chitta.

This dichotomy is not all that alien to the Western experience. Compare, for example, this admission of Thoreau's: "I only know myself as a human entity; the scene, so to speak, of thoughts and affections; and am sensible of a certain doubleness by which I can stand as remote from myself as from another. However intense my experience, I am conscious of the presence and criticism of a part of me, which, as it were, is not a part of me, but spectator, sharing no experience, but taking note of it; and that is no more I than it is you."[8]

Purusha—Thoreau's "spectator"—is that faculty in us whose role is to observe, to bear witness. All other functions of "mind" belong to chitta, which is the instrument or agent of purusha. Both are essential, but it is purusha which is at the center of our being. When there is chitta-vrtti nirodha, purusha can see clearly, and what we do is likely to turn out well. But when chitta is disturbed, purusha becomes temporarily obscured, and our action loses some of its integrity (I.3-4).

After noting that the adjuncts to a tranquil mind are assiduousness and equanimity (I.12-16), Patanjali distinguishes two levels of samadhi. One is the outcome of reflection on the form and nature of the object; there is a sense of joy in discovery and an awareness of oneself as discoverer. Samadhi may also exist wherein even the awareness of oneself disappears (I.17-18). Progress in Yoga requires dedication, strength of purpose, and intelligence. Samadhi and the insight it engenders become a feature in our experience. (I.19-22).

The aspirant in Yoga may also take support from the concept of *īshwara*. Ishwara is described as the consummate purusha, free from imperfections and the cycle of actions and consequences, infinitely knowing, and unbounded by time. Meditating on ishwara may soothe us and give us an intimation of possibilities beyond our present powers (I.23-29).

Naturally there are obstacles along the path to Yoga. These are enumerated as: disease, sluggishness, doubt, heedlessness, exhaustion, indulgence, delusion, inability to attain a further stage, and inability to maintain a stage already reached. These obstacles, and the confusion or distraction often responsible for them, show up in anxiety, unhappiness, and unsteadiness of body and breath. At such times it is helpful to hold fast to some tried-and-true principle—be it a religious or intellectual formulation, or a calming activity of any sort (I.30-32).

Patanjali suggests various practices by which the chitta may be made less confused and more clear (I.33-39), such as:

1. Cultivating good will toward happy persons, compassion toward suffering, gladness toward virtue, and disdain toward vice.
2. Watching the movement of the breath.
3. Emulating magnanimous individuals.
4. Pondering the phenomena of dreaming and sleeping.
5. Any other type of meditation or appropriate technique (dhyana).

Patanjali now returns to the qualities of samadhi, and offers us a simile. The chitta without distractions is likened to a polished crystal. Placed against a surface, it assumes the coloration of that surface and can scarcely be detected as a separate entity. If we take the eye to be purusha, the glass to be chitta, and the colored surface to be the object, we can understand how the apprehending or reflecting function of chitta becomes less and less distinguishable from the object itself, as chitta loses its opacity. The perceiver and the act of perceiving become one with the perceived (I.41).

Samadhi becomes progressively refined as the object of contemplation becomes more subtle, and as the tendency of the mind to verbalize, rationalize, and fabricate is lessened. In propor-

tion as we bring memory to bear, our perception of the present object is tainted; we are seeing what *was*, more than what *is*. If perception could be purified of prior impressions, each object would be seen for what it is intrinsically. The less our perception is veiled by preconception, the more transparent is chitta, the more prominent is purusha, and the more complete the resulting understanding.

Ultimately, the only reliable knowledge is that which we experience directly; inference and testimony are not as trustworthy. The impression left by a direct perception works to inhibit the formation of fallacious impressions. Samadhi culminates—logically if not demonstrably—when even the relatively pure impressions cease to be formed, and knowledge is perfect (I.42-51).

What Yoga calls samadhi is by no means the monopoly of Oriental experience. In America, it has been given eloquent expression by Thoreau, as well as by more recent authors. See, for example, Annie Dillard's *Pilgrim at Tinker Creek*,[9] and Robert M. Pirsig's *Zen and the Art of Motorcycle Maintenance: An Inquiry into Values*.[10]

THE TREADMILL

In Part II of the Yoga Sutra, Patanjali tries to analyze why samadhi is not as simple as it sounds. He isolates five internal forces that work to disturb our minds and corrupt our actions. Any one of these five *kleshas* may preponderate—the others being temporarily concealed—or they may all be more or less attenuated. At best, they remain potential, as seeds awaiting the right conditions for sprouting.

Foremost among the kleshas is *avidyā*, which implies something more than any of the words by which it is usually translated: "ignorance, misapprehension, nescience, misconception." Avidya consists in mistaking the transitory for the perm-anent, the impure for the pure, the painful for the pleasurable, and chitta for purusha. It is the field from which grow the other four kleshas (II.3-5).

After avidya comes the feeling of "I am." With-out a sense of self we cannot operate. Where we get into trouble is in believing that the active "I," the personality with which we clothe ourselves, possesses sovereign power; when in fact it shares the power with what we have called purusha (II.6).

The third and fourth kleshas form a pair: yearning after pleasure, and avoidance of pain. Pleasure and pain, in all their manifestations, are great motivators. We instinctively (often against our better judgment), turn toward that which has given us pleasure, and away from that which has caused us pain. Depending on the degree of pleasure or pain, these feelings will vary in inten-sity anywhere from like and dislike to obsession and loathing. If hate can be a klesha, so can love, when it is not tempered by clear thinking (II.7-8).

The last of the kleshas is the will to live, which is tantamount to the fear of loss—whether of ourselves or of that to which we are attached. This one is particularly tenacious—inborn, no doubt—and persists even in the wise. Our thoughts and actions generate fears; then those fears entrap us (II.9).

The danger in the kleshas is that they are self-aggrandizing. Actions motivated by klesha leave a residue, which adds to our store of klesha and prejudices future action. We cannot cease acting, but we can strive to reduce klesha (II.10-14). It is questionable, however, whether the kleshas can be eliminated altogether. The sensitive person, therefore, remains a little wary even when things seem to be going well.

In fact, the usual state of affairs is not joy at all, but rather what is called *duhkha*. The opposite of *sukha*, which we shall encounter a little later,

duhkha can be defined as "pain, hardship, misery, suffering, discomfort, distress, anxiety." It may be sensed physically, or it may be exclusively in the mind—an uneasiness or tension, or a feeling that our options are restricted or our freedom com-promised. Duhkha may be imposed on us by an outside agency, or we may bring it on ourselves. Even if we could prevent the latter kind, we would still have to contend with the former. Perhaps the best we can do is to try to avoid, or at least be prepared for, the duhkha that has not yet ar-rived (II.15-16).

Duhkha is a by-product of avidya, which, as we have seen, is a faulty grasp of reality, especially as regards the nature of the self. We tend to iden-tify with chitta, but chitta is not the whole story. Chitta exists to serve purusha. Insofar as we recognize the distinction between them, our avidya is lessened, and with it our duhkha (II.27.27).

GETTING THERE FROM HERE

The reciprocal relationship between action and klesha explains why an unusual type of action is required—one which is not deliberate or tied to the past. If we would improve the quality of action we must allow for a little *reflection*. The true moment of Yoga is the pause *before* action. (Fitting it is that the entire Bhagavad Gita is transmitted to Arjuna in the moment before he charges into battle—while time obligingly stands still!) It is before we begin acting that we are most clear. Action coming after reflection is therefore less likely to turn out wrong.

What we have called "reflection"—in transla-tion of *dhyāna*—is customarily referred to as "meditation"; but use of the latter word involves us in semantic difficulties. Is meditation, for exam-ple, a conscious thinking about something—or what happens in an unguarded moment when we are *not* consciously thinking? Can it be practiced—

or must it be spontaneous? Has the word (which is from the Latin), the same implications in Eastern as in Western usage? A typical dictionary definition of meditation is "exercising the mind in contemplation." Dhyana, however, may also refer to the unpremeditated product of that exercise; so it is not strictly synonymous with meditation.

For Patanjali, Yoga resides not only in dhyana-samadhi, but in the *procedure* employed to encourage that state. Part II of the Yoga Sutra (subtitled "On Practice") recommends first the "Yoga of Action." (*Kriyā Yoga;* II.1-2) intended to give us an intimation of samadhi and weaken the kleshas; then the more ambitious and inclusive "Eight-Part Yoga" (*Aṣhṭāṅga Yoga;* II.28-29).

However helpful solitary meditation may be, it must not be at odds with the lives of relation we necessarily lead. Accordingly, the Eight-Part Yoga rests on principles of right conduct. These are ten in number, and are divided into two groups, called *yama* and *niyama* (II.30-45).

In the first group are:

1. Kindness, harmlessness (*ahimsā*).
2. Truthfulness (*satya*).
3. Non-stealing, honesty (*asteya*).
4. Continence; moderation in sensual desires (*brahmacharya*).
5. Absence of greed; non-possessiveness (*aparigraha*).

In the second group are:

6. Purity, cleanliness (*shaucha*].
7. Contentment, tranquility (*santoṣha*).
8. Self-discipline, austerity; keeping oneself fit (*tapas*).
9. Study, introspection, intellectual earnestness (*swādhyāya*).
10. Humility in action; acknowledging a higher principle (*Īshwara praṇidhāna*).

(Nos. 8-10 also appear in II.1 as the Yoga of Action.)

It must not be assumed that yama and niyama have to be mastered before one can proceed in Yoga. In fact, they can never be mastered, but continue to provide a standard of behavior for practitioners at all levels.

By the time the Yoga Sutra was composed, Yoga had become far more than a technique for achieving magical powers or release from worldly bondage. It had matured into a comprehensive approach to life, requiring a solid foundation in interpersonal morality. Teachers of Yoga had also become convinced that, far from being irrelevant or inimical, *physical fitness* is an impetus to spiritual progress. With "disciplined activity" extended to the physical as well as psychic level, the basis was laid for a system of integrated physico-mental training with wide application. Meditation and liberation are admirable objectives, but they are extraordinarily elusive. To have an experience of these, most persons need a down-to-earth preliminary technique.

Thus, according to Yoga, lofty aspiration is not enough. Even right conduct is not enough. We must also learn to understand ourselves as physical creatures. We must become more stable, more relaxed, more sure of ourselves. An invaluable preparation for dhyana, therefore is *āsana*.

WHAT IS ASANA?

This word, by now familiar to Westerners, comes from the verb "to sit." *Āsana* literally means "sitting"—and by extension, "remaining, staying, position, posture." It is described quite well by this modern definition of "posture": "an unmoving but dynamic position of the body, maintained by neuromuscular activity."[11] However, in its earliest appearances in texts on Yoga, asana did indeed mean "sitting"; one had to sit still in order to meditate.

In the course of time, yogins began to experiment with postures other than those facilitating meditation. Other seated postures were probably tried first, after which it must have seemed logical to practice lying, inverted, and standing postures. What made these exercises original was the emphasis on motionlessness in the pose, borrowed from the physical stillness characteristic of seated meditation. The challenge was to transfer the calmness and alertness of the meditative attitude to postures requiring altogether different muscular control. A new branch of Yoga arose, complete with authoritative inventories of the various asanas, together with instructions and alleged benefits (sometimes in fanciful or cryptic language). Among such texts which have come down to us are the *Haṭha Yoga Pradīpikā*, *Shiva Samhitā*, *Gheraṇḍa Samhitā*, and *Yoga Yājñavalkya*.

A considerable number of asanas must have been known to Patanjali, so it may seem surprising that, in setting forth the classic doctrine of Yoga, he chose not to refer to any by name. Even more disconcerting to the modern reader, accustomed to find asanas fleshing out every book on yoga, is the discovery that Patanjali devotes a mere three sutras to the consideration of asana (Part II, sutras 46-48). Of these, the second and third require a good deal of interpretation, but the first is crystal clear and a miracle of conciseness. Its two simple adjectives say everything essential about asana: *Sthira-sukham āsanam*.

Sthira can be defined as "firm, strong, motionless, steady, sustained."

Sukha means "comfortable, pleasant, agreeable, easy."

Āsana, therefore, is that which is *both sthira and sukha*. Tense rigidity is not asana, nor is flaccid repose. Asana is the conjunction of two qualities normally thought to be contradictory.

Having made this point, Patanjali does not go on to recommend specific asanas; that is left to other writers and teachers. What interests Patanjali is not so much the variety of postures the human body can assume as the attributes any posture must possess if it is to be truly termed "āsana."

Thus, *Padmāsana* (Lotus) may be an asana by name, but it is not really functioning as an asana unless you are both steady and comfortable. There is an important lesson here, which we shall have ample occasion to cite in subsequent chapters.

ASANA AND MEDITATION

Although his definition applies equally well to all conceivable postures, Patanjali probably had seated asanas in mind. The subject of the Yoga Sutra is mental poise, and sitting was known empirically as the physical position most conducive to its achievement.

Fundamental as they are, seated asanas are among the most difficult. Just see how long you can sit in any posture without tiring! Unless you have been practicing for many months, you will soon feel fatigue in your back, hips, or legs; you will start to squirm, and will want to change position.

Discomfort in sitting is less a racial than a cultural legacy. As people migrated to colder climates where sitting on the ground was no longer feasible, chairs became more than a status symbol. Our ancestors had somehow managed to support their own backs, but we have relinquished that responsibility to our chairs—most of which are designed so that we can't sit straight in them even if we want to.

It is axiomatic in Yoga that the activity of the mind reflects the attitude of the body. In order to sustain any high-quality mind work we must be able effortlessly to sustain an erect position. As long as our posture is fitful our brilliance will be too. We can maintain an erect vertebral column in postures other than seated, and we can be comfortable for extended periods in other postures. But only seated can we remain for long both comfortable and firm. It is for this reason that Yoga prizes the seated asanas. And it is largely to prepare the body for sitting still that we have recourse to the other classes of asanas: standing, supine, prone, inverted, etc.

Though the goal of asana is stillness, it is often helpful to incorporate controlled movement within asanas of all classes. The question of stillness versus movement will be taken up in the chapters to follow.

If asana is an aid to dhyana, so is it a *model* for dhyana. Indeed, sthira-sukha is as good a definition of mental as of physical poise. A mind that is steady yet relaxed is surely what we all desire. If the body is, to some extent, a reflection or counterpart of the mind, then attention to the body should teach us a great deal about our inner selves and the way we live our lives. Asana is not only a preparation for meditation; it is itself a profound meditation.

Practicing asanas requires, to begin with, that we observe our physical condition. Doing so is not easy; it takes considerable sensitivity to notice the body's signals. In life we often have to wait a long time before appreciating the full effects of insensitive actions. In asana we know right away. Presumably, prompt feedback promotes quicker learning and increased sensitivity.

And when we observe our physical condition, what do we see? For one thing, we see that each of us is unique and never quite the same as the last time we looked. With the needs and capacities of the body always changing, it becomes harder to think of personality as something unchanging.

Yet beneath our shifting physical states we can sense a consistency, a continuity, an identity. As different as we are from day to day, we are never completely different. Something in us abides—if only to keep track of that part of us which is changeable.

Examining our physical selves, we inevitably confront certain resistances, certain inhibitions. We may be stiff, or lazy, or weak, or tense, or restless, or uncoordinated. If in combating such tendencies we are rash, we can get hurt or frustrated. On the other hand, if we opt to ignore them, they may become even greater impediments. Our minds too have their handicaps; these must be acknowledged and dealt with if we are to grow emotionally. Though hard on the ego, daily contact with our limitations may at least make us more tolerant of the limitations of others.

Resistances and inhibitions are not easily overcome. They are ingrained and are being continually reinforced. Asanas show us to what extent our bodies are conditioned: we can move in certain ways but not in others; we can stay in certain positions but not in others. Just so, the mind is restricted by its conditioning. We are creatures of habit. Habits themselves are not intrinsically harmful; we could not function if our every action had to be thought out in all its details. The danger is in allowing habits to outlive their usefulness. Even the best of them periodically need to be reevaluated, if not replaced. If our behavior is mostly determined by our genes, our environment, and our conditioning, there is all the more reason to exercise what little free will remains to us.

As the practice of asanas quickly shows us, it is enormously difficult to counteract the effects of conditioning. It takes time, patience, and effort. Recognizing a problem is a first vital step, but it must be followed by activity—concerted and prolonged. There is no substitute for work—so long as we work intelligently. We must exercise what needs to be exercised, and in a suitable manner. Too little effort gets us nowhere; too much effort can break us.

Asanas also remind us that the goal toward which we direct our effort is ultimately less important than the effort itself. If we stop striving once we attain our goal, what is to prevent us from slipping back? The only solution is to find a new goal sufficiently pertinent to spur a continuing effort. Even if we fail to achieve our initial goal we can learn from the attempt. In trying unsuccessfully to do A, I may discover that I should be doing B. Then I can shift my direction and work on B. Whereas practicing without even a tentative goal I might never have realized my need for B. What at first we think we need is not always what we really need. But the more we get to know ourselves, the more obvious are the goals we should be striving for. Asana is an excellent means for getting to know ourselves better.

Accepting our limitations, setting feasible goals, and working steadily, it is not long before we detect some improvement. Any physical improvement is already an aid to emotional well-being—though it has a deeper value in suggesting that improvement may also be possible in other, unsuspected areas. Brief and painful as it is, life can be exhilarating when we feel we are moving forward. Without this feeling, life becomes tedious if not unbearable. Not only must we improve; we must see the improvement. Asanas can help us do both.

ASANA AND WELL-BEING

The foregoing rationale for Yoga exercise may seem excessively philosophical. In fact, you need not do asanas for the reasons we have given. You can approach them as you would any other type of exercise, and you can expect results at least as favorable.

The strictly physiological benefits of exercise are many and have been well-established. Activity improves motor abilities, muscle tone, circulatory and respiratory efficiency, body posture, digestion and assimilation, elimination of toxins, and resistance to disease. It gives you more energy, makes you more alert, helps you sleep soundly, makes you feel and look better, and may lengthen your life.

What is less well-established is the need for *violent* exercise. The Occidental exercise tradition derives in part from military training, and is biased toward competition and the attainment of ever higher performance levels. It puts a premium on all-out effort and does not always lead to optimum health. Without wishing to indict Western physical education, we simply suggest that exercise need not be violent in order to serve its basic purpose. Though comparatively mild, asanas—done regularly—may be more than adequate.

You can do asanas in addition to other physical activities, as a preparation for other activities, or as an alternative to other activities.

Asanas can help keep you in good overall health. You can also use them selectively to loosen or strengthen any part of the body. Tight muscles and stiff joints respond well to asana practice, as do muscles that are underdeveloped or easily fatigued. Certain visceral malfunctions can be helped by asanas. Asanas can reduce nervous tension as well as physical tension.

Health can be measured by certain universal parameters; *fitness* relates to your individual needs. If your work is physically exhausting, you don't need an exercise that will tire you even more. If your work is sedentary, you need a type of exercise which will give you a good workout, yet enable you to be more comfortable reading and writing for hours at a time. If you must be on your feet a lot, you need an exercise which will both compensate for the negative effects of standing, and allow you more comfortably to stand for long periods. When you are robust your exercise can be vigorous; when you are convalescing it should be gentle. Asanas can be adapted to all these needs.

All thoroughgoing exercise systems are concerned not only with muscles, but with the heart and lungs—broadly, the *circulo-respiratory* system. Whereas some types of exercise work on circulo-respiratory endurance by speeding up the breathing and heart rates to near-maximum levels, Yoga strengthens the heart and lungs chiefly by slowing down and deepening the breath. Conscious breathing can be a vital component of asana practice and is the substance of *pranayama*.

Systems of exercise must also make adequate provision for *relaxation*. Muscles can be trained to do more work, but if they are not taught also to relax they will not perform to capacity. "In fact, muscle fibres work most efficiently in terms of endurance when contraction and relaxation alternate with a sufficiently long relaxation period to clear the lactic acid between contractions. Endurance is achieved by rotating the work load around different motor units, allowing some to relax while others work."[12] This phenomenon accounts for the importance given in Yoga to compensatory stretching and frequent resting.

Muscles are linked to nerves. When stimulated by an attached motor neuron, the fibers of a muscle contract. Complex movements require innervation of many muscles. New contractions are constantly being triggered, while tired muscle fibers are allowed a brief rest. At the same time, the "stretch reflex" is causing contractions in the antagonist muscle groups.

Nerve impulses emanate from control centers in the spinal cord and brain. Impulse patterns productive of often-repeated muscular contractions are codified to permit automatic recall. In other words, subconscious motor habits are always being formed, based on the capabilities of the local muscles. Such conditioning is obviously an advantage, but can also be a curse when, because of physiological imbalances, the muscle combinations employed are not the best ones.

Asanas, in bringing conscious attention to muscular activity, can redirect the nerve impulses along more desirable pathways, resulting in altered and improved reflexes and habits.

Thus, via muscles and nerves, we are back to the mind—where we started from! Psychological and physiological justifications for practicing Yoga, though proceeding in opposite directions, inevitably bump into one another. This, of course, is what makes Yoga unique. Other philosophical systems have explored the same mental territory; other exercise systems have dealt with the same physical needs. But the former have usually ignored the body and the latter the mind. In Yoga, what counts is the harmony between the two. Mind and body must not function at the expense of one another.

All along we have been very serious. But there is also another aspect to the picture: Yoga as *play*. We have said that Yoga entails effort, but good work is invariably a joy as well. Spending time in different postures and experiencing new ones should be fun. Attentiveness may be necessary for Yoga, but solemnity is not. In making you healthier and more fit, your practice will also make you happier.

2

QUESTIONS AND ANSWERS

When I was new to Yoga I naturally had my share of questions. As I began to practice, still more occurred to me which had to do with various aspects of the subject. I have since learned that such questions are asked at some point by almost everyone involved with Yoga. The questions are urgent and need to be answered before too much confusion arises. For this reason I have grouped together some of the more important ones in this chapter, along with the answers I now would give, based on my own experience and study.

Q: How often should I practice Yoga?

A: As often as you like. If you want to make progress you will have to practice fairly often, but an occasional session is better than none at all. Continuity is important; practicing three times a week regularly will probably accomplish more than six times one week and only once the next.

That doesn't mean you have to become compulsive about Yoga. If you have to skip your practice now and then, there is no harm done. An occasional holiday from Yoga may give you a fresh perspective on your practice.

Q: For how long should I practice?

A: Ideally, for at least an hour every day; it takes time to do a balanced, complete routine. However, shorter practice sessions are also worthwhile. You can do a lot in half an hour if you make

a good choice of exercises. What counts is not so much clock time as the experience of a distinctive physico-mental state. But a certain amount of time is needed in order to ease yourself into and out of that state.

With experience, you will be able to chart a Yoga course that will fit comfortably into the time you have to spare. Keep in mind that, as a general rule, it is better to do a few asanas thoughtfully than a whole series in haste. And you should always allow time for resting, especially at the end of your practice.

Q: Will I need to spend more time practicing as I learn more exercises?

A: No. Each practice session consists of a selection from among the exercises you know. On a given day you need do only what you feel will be most beneficial. The more you know, the more abundant is the store from which you can choose.

You may find, in fact, that the more advanced you become, the fewer asanas you need to do in any one practice. You will be doing them more slowly and getting deeper effects.

Q: When is the best time to practice?

A: Whenever is most convenient. It should be a time when you can allow yourself to relax and when you are least likely to be disturbed by others. Some people prefer to practice first thing in the morning, some during lunch break, some after finishing work, some before retiring at night.

Early in the morning the body is rested, the stomach empty, and the mind not yet preoccupied. But the joints are relatively stiff and the muscles slack, due to inactivity and lowered body temperature. Consequently you will have to devote more attention to warming up. Don't expect your body to be as limber as it would be later in the day.

Yoga may be a nice way to break up the working day, assuming you can find a good place to practice, but if you try to squeeze it into a short space before lunch you may find yourself rushing through the asanas without breathing deeply or allowing yourself sufficient rest—not to mention bolting your food in the few minutes remaining.

Late afternoon may be the ideal time, since body and mind tend to be at low ebb after a day's work. Even a short practice should relax you for dinner and restore your energy for the evening's activities. It is probably the safest time of day to exercise, especially if you have been leading a sedentary life. However, if family or other responsibilities prevent you from doing Yoga at this time, you can surely find another. Many persons with children to care for, for example, find the best period to be late morning, while the children are at school or playing.

There are conflicting opinions about practicing Yoga before bedtime. Some people find that it tires and relaxes them thoroughly, releasing stored-up tension and permitting them to sleep easily and well. Others feel that Yoga at night gives them a belated surge of energy and delays falling asleep.

There is one stipulation, however, about practice time: Never do Yoga on a full stomach. For two to three hours after a meal the body is busily engaged in digestion. Physical exercise during this time draws blood to the muscles and limbs, inter-

fering with blood flow to the stomach. Since in Yoga we want to stretch the muscles deeply and massage the inner organs, it is best to wait until digestion in the stomach has been substantially completed. Walking or other light activity a short while after a meal does not hinder digestion, and may allow you to practice Yoga sooner than if you merely sat or reclined for a few hours. Of course, after a snack or a beverage you need not wait three hours before doing Yoga; you can start as soon as you feel light.

Otherwise there are no rules about when to practice. You will have to experiment and decide which time suits you best. If it is possible for you to reserve the same hour every day (or every other day) for Yoga, you may find it easier to be regular in your practice.

Q: What should I wear to practice Yoga?

A: Wear as little as comfort and decorum demand. Protection is essential in cold climates, but clothing should not inhibit you from bending and stretching to your fullest extent. Loose-fitting shorts, pyjamas, or swimming attire are fine for warm environments; sweatshirt or pullover, and sweat pants or baggy trousers for cold. Many people like to wear leotards for Yoga; others feel that they interfere with perspiration. Suit yourself!

Q: What equipment will I need?

A: All you need is a mat: something thicker than a folded towel or blanket, but not so soft as a foam rubber pad. A cotton carpet is ideal if you can get one. If not, a section of wool or acrylic carpeting will do, though you may want to lay a cotton cloth or towel over it. The mat should be only thick enough to cushion your bones. It should not, like a mattress, fill in the curves in your spinal column. A mattress is fine for sleeping, but in Yoga you want to stay awake and attentive even while you relax.

For practicing inverted postures you will need added padding, since the skull, neck, and shoulders are not naturally cushioned to bear the full weight of the body.

Further, you may want to have on hand some common "props," such as a pillow or a book. These can be used to simplify or intensify asanas as need be.

Q: Does it matter where I do my practice?

A: Try to practice in a room you like being in, which is well ventilated but not cold or drafty. It should not contain too many objects to distract you, though it need not be bare as a prison cell. If you are happiest and most relaxed surrounded by books, paintings, plants, furniture, and familiar objects, you can try doing your Yoga there as well. See how it goes. Just make sure you have plenty of room to move about in, and space enough for your mat.

Q: Should I do any warm-ups before starting my Yoga practice?

A: The best way to warm up for Yoga is with Yoga. In fact, Yoga asanas can be an excellent warm-up for other physical activities. Rather than starting with leg pumping or arm swinging, we try in Yoga to increase circulation to the extremities and superficial muscles by deepening the breath. It is prudent not to risk straining the joints while the body is still cold, though some conventional warm-ups do just that. The way warm-ups function in Yoga will be illustrated in subsequent chapters.

If you tend to be stiff, or if the room in which you practice is chilly, it is a good idea to take a hot bath or shower beforehand.

Q: I know quite a few postures. Does it make any difference in what order I do them?

A: Definitely. You have only to mix up a series of postures to feel how different is their effect—both individually and cumulatively. The effect of a posture cannot be predicted apart from its context, and depends on a variety of factors. We shall go into these later.

Q: Is it advisable to do Yoga when one is preoccupied or under emotional stress?

A: Why not? It is true that Yoga has to do with concentration, but it is not true that to do Yoga you must have concentration to start with. Slow movements, gentle stretching, and deep breathing often help to relax and stabilize the mind. Thus Yoga may be most useful to you precisely when you feel too upset or distracted to practice.

Q: I seem to have a very stiff body. I couldn't dream of ever doing most of the postures I've seen. Am I right in assuming that Yoga is not for me?

A: If the postures you have seen are not presently feasible for you, it may be possible to simplify them. Some postures which you have not seen may also be of use. But if you are very stiff it is well to proceed slowly—preferably under the supervision of a good teacher.

Q: Must I expect a certain amount of pain from the practice of asanas?

A: Pain is not an indication that the body is improving; it is a setback to improvement. Pain may reveal the presence of a stiff or weak area, but it proves that you have gone too far in exercising it. Recuperation from the strain behind the pain will take time, so what do you gain?

Courting pain is also bad psychology. The healthy response to pain is aversion to that which occasioned it. If your pain is the result of Yoga, how long are you likely to continue practicing? Thus pain is not to be expected; it is to be forestalled. There is enough pain in life already without Yoga contributing more. We may occasionally experience some accidental soreness despite our best efforts; but if your asana practice regularly gives you pain, something about it is wrong.

Q: Standing on the head seems to me a particularly perverse practice. Why does Yoga set such great store by it?

A: If standing on the head is unnatural, it is at least a lot healthier than many of the other unnatural things we do all the time. Nevertheless, your skepticism is warranted. Whatever its theoretical advantages, this pose is not advisable for many persons. The pros and cons, as well as the technique, of Headstand are discussed in Chapter 7.

Q: Will Yoga interfere with participation in sports?

A: Why should it? If anything, Yoga will increase your stamina and lessen the risk of strained joints or pulled muscles.

Q: What about eye exercise?

A: Various eye exercises have been associated with Yoga. Your teacher may be able to show you some which will be of use to you.

Be careful with your eyes; they take a lot of abuse. You may think you should be exercising them when what they most need is rest. You might try "palming" them from time to time. This involves warming the hands and cupping them gently over the eye sockets so that no light enters between the fingers. Close your eyes, let them relax, and try to imagine total blackness. Palming can be practiced in a seated posture accompanied by Yoga breathing.

Q: If I practice Yoga regularly will I need to sleep less?

A: Very likely. Inasmuch as it relaxes the mind and speeds removal of toxins from body tissues, a regular practice of Yoga may enable you to manage with less sleep. Almost certainly, you will fall asleep more easily and sleep more soundly. Whether or not it actually reduces the number of hours you spend sleeping, Yoga should make you more wakeful and energetic the rest of the time—when you *don't* want to be sleeping.

Q: Is it true Yoga will help me lose weight?

A: Your weight depends on many factors, not all of which are under your control. You can't change your genetic inheritance, your body type, or your basic personality, but you can do something about your eating habits and activity level. Other things being equal, if you take in fewer calories than you burn up, you will lose weight. So you must either eat less (of high-caloric foods) or work more.

In terms of calories burned, Yoga cannot compete with conventional exercise. However, it is questionable whether heavy exercise is all that efficient as a means to lose weight. Such effect as it has may be neutralized by an exaggerated appetite afterward. Yoga will not exhaust you but will help to regularize your body's metabolism. It can also counteract the glandular dysfunctions that are sometimes the latent cause of obesity. You may find your appetite becoming a more reliable index of needed caloric intake.

Yoga feels best when the stomach is light. If you enjoy practicing Yoga you will thus have positive reinforcement for eating less heavily and less frequently. It would be interesting to see test results of long-term weight fluctuations among practitioners of Yoga who were overweight to begin with.

No one can guarantee that you will lose weight by practicing Yoga. You might even gain. Not everybody needs to weigh less; you may be too thin or too flabby. You can tell whether a weight gain is desirable by noting its concomitant symptoms. Do you feel well? Are you energetic? Do you have a healthy appetite? Are you sleeping soundly? If you answer yes to all of these, the extra weight is probably good for you.

Q: I've been told that I have high blood pressure. Is it safe for me to do Yoga?

A: High blood pressure need not rule out Yoga, provided you have your doctor's approval. Practiced sensibly, Yoga may even help to bring your pressure down.

Q: Can Yoga help me quit smoking?

A: Smoking and Yoga are mutually exclusive in a profound sense. You cannot long continue to care for your body and abuse it at the same time. Guilt feelings are unpleasant; sooner or later something has to give. If Yoga has set up in you a healthful habit, as pleasurable in its own way as smoking, it will gradually weaken the unhealthy habit. At some point there will be a stand-off. It may be a painful period. Whichever habit represents the stronger urge will prevail. If you still want to smoke, Yoga may be the casualty. But if by the critical period you have come to love Yoga, you will quit smoking, and very likely quit for good.

Q: Why does Yoga advocate conscious breath control? I've read that since breathing is an involuntary function it shouldn't be tampered with.

A: Breathing is only partly involuntary, and we tamper with it all the time. Every cigarette puff, every breath in a stuffy room or a big city—everything we do to weaken the defenses of our respiratory apparatus proves the effectiveness of voluntary intervention. In Yoga at least we intervene for positive effects. See Chapter 6.

Q: Isn't holding the breath dangerous?

A: It can be. But practiced with moderation and care, under your teacher's supervision, breath holding is one of the most effective techniques of Yoga. Only use a little common sense; you can overdose even on vitamins. Chapter 8 explains the use of breath holding in Yoga.

Q: Should a pregnant woman refrain from practicing Yoga?

A: How much Yoga she should do is largely a function of her state of fitness prior to pregnancy. If she had been practicing Yoga regularly she can continue—gradually simplifying her practice as necessary. Certain postures may have to be abandoned, but Yoga breathing can be very helpful. A pregnant woman with a background in Yoga or athletics should begin Yoga only under expert supervision, and with her doctor's approval.

Q: The Yoga classes I've observed consist mostly of women. Is Yoga not as useful for men?

A: There is no reason why it should not be. In India, Yoga was for centuries one of the most respected pursuits a man could have. The needs of men and women may not be identical, but both sexes can benefit from the practice of Yoga.

Q: Is Yoga good for children?

A: Yes, so long as it is adapted to their special needs. Asanas can be used to increase strength as well as suppleness. Teaching Yoga to children involves considerable responsibility, and presupposes a thorough training.

Q: Is Yoga safe for the elderly?

A: A scaled-down course of movements derived from Yoga asanas can benefit elderly persons. Naturally, all extreme stretches and strenuous movements must be avoided, and suitable modifications made for persons with special handicaps. Stiffness in the spinal column and joints will probably rule out inversion, back bending, and most floor sitting. Much can be done, however, while seated on a chair. Cushions or other props may facilitate supine and standing poses. An ingenious Yoga teacher could conceivably accomplish a great deal with elderly persons, even the least ambulatory among them.

As in other cases of physical disability, it is through breathing that Yoga may be of most help to the aged and infirm. Breathing is vital, everyone does it, and everyone can learn to do it better—

irrespective of age. Improved breathing habits may result in functional improvements not otherwise attainable.

If you have been practicing Yoga since middle age, the question of safety hardly arises. You can continue practicing indefinitely, although little by little you will have to give up the more extreme postures. To a great extent, Yoga will immunize you from the ravages of time. Degeneration of the viscera and stiffening of the joints will be retarded, and you will feel younger longer.

Q: Must I give up meat in order to benefit from Yoga?

A: No. The closest Yoga comes to prohibiting meat is in the concept of *ahimsa*, which literally means "non-harming." You do have to harm an animal in order to eat it, but you may be harming yourself, psychologically as well as physically, by giving up the food your body is used to, without first giving deep thought. Some persuasive arguments have been advanced for adopting a vegetarian diet, but total abstention from meat is certainly not a precondition for practicing Yoga.

Q: What about fasting?

A: Fasting is an extreme therapy which may be appropriate in certain extreme conditions; it is not a part of Yoga practice. Texts on Yoga counsel moderation in all things, including diet.

Q: Is it true that a serious practitioner of Yoga must refrain from sexual activity?

A: No. Yoga is not anti-life, and sex is a vital part of the life process. If celibacy causes you psychic damage, how can it help you to be a better person? The controversial word *brahmacharya* doesn't mean "celibacy" in the strict sense. It is more a concern to keep sensual desires from getting so out of hand that they diminish rather than enhance the joy of living.

Q: Why haven't you mentioned *kuṇḍalinī* and the *chakras*?

A: Although these concepts figure prominently in certain branches of the Yogic tradition, they are not treated in the Yoga Sutra. Since they have also not been a part of this writer's experience they are not discussed in this book.

Q: What is meant by the term "Hatha Yoga"?

A: The word *hatha* seems to imply some sort of vehement physical practice, but the origins of Hatha Yoga are obscure. It must have meant more than simply "asana and pranayama," though it is sometimes used nowadays in this sense. The term is not employed in the Yoga Sutra, and we shall do without it here.

Q: How does Yoga differ from Transcendental Meditation?

A: Transcendental Meditation is a simplified version of traditional Yogic meditation. Physiological tests have shown it to be effective in producing a state of deep relaxation. Other tests have proved that a similar state results from the practice of Yoga.

TM purposely dispenses with the physical conditioning which is so important in Yoga. Proponents of Yoga argue that the benefits of practicing asana and pranayama are more lasting than those deriving from TM alone. In fact, TM also values asana and pranayama, but introduces them only in the advanced course.

Q: My work requires me to be very creative. If it makes the mind quiet, isn't Yoga inimical to creativity?

A: Yoga may quiet the mind; it does not annihilate it. The object of Yoga is not to neutralize your personality, but to make your thought and action more harmonious and confident. If creativity is something genuine, if it comes from the depths of your being, shouldn't it be enhanced by any practice which puts you at ease and in touch with yourself?

Q: Is it true that yogis acquire supernormal powers?

A: I'll have to pass on this question. Who is a "yogi"? And where do you draw the line between normal and supernormal powers? This whole area makes me uncomfortable.

The Yoga Sutra concedes that supernormal powers may accrue to exceptional individuals at an advanced stage of concentration. It also warns that such powers, if indulged in, can themselves become obstacles to mental clarity. It is as if they were granted, not as a reward, but to test the yogin's ability to remain undeterred by them.

Q: I know that in India people have traditionally learned Yoga from a guru. Is it really necessary nowadays to have a teacher? Can't one learn just as well from books, cassettes, and television programs?

A: At the time the guru system evolved, the only way knowledge and experience could be preserved was by oral transmission. Since then there has been a revolution in the acquisition, storage, and dissemination of information. Nostalgia for a simpler life is understandable, but as long as books, tape, and TV are here to stay, we would be foolish not to exploit them for the great good they can do.

The media can teach us many things, but when it comes to Yoga their advantage is less evident. As long as individuals remain so different from one another, Yoga cannot successfully be prepackaged. Books, cassettes, or TV can teach you the rudiments of asanas, but not the subtlety with which they can be adapted to your personal needs. To appreciate Yoga at this level, you must have a guide who can get to know you as an individual and observe your practice.

Q: There are so many varieties of Yoga being offered. How can I choose between them? How can I judge the qualifications of a Yoga teacher?

A: It is hard to choose among unknowns. Be glad at least that you have a choice of approaches and instructors. Since the subject of Yoga comprises such enormous variety and divergence, it would be difficult to establish objective standards by which to assess the qualifications of prospective teachers. There are different kinds of Yoga for different people. Shop around. Trust your instincts and misgivings. What do the qualifications of a Yoga teacher amount to, if not the ability to make Yoga meaningful and enjoyable for you?

Q: Should I sign up for a Yoga class even if I won't have time to practice at home?

A: Why not? Sometimes it is good to start slowly. See whether Yoga interests you before you make a commitment to it.

Practicing between classes will allow you to assimilate what you have learned and make more rapid progress. But if you have forgotten the sequence of the poses or are not sure you are executing them correctly, it is better to wait until you can resolve your doubts at the next class meeting.

If you feel good doing Yoga you may manage to find time to do a few of your favorite poses at home, even without being able to set aside a regular practice period.

Q: I've never considered taking private lessons. Is there any reason why I should?

A: A group class may be more practical, especially if you have not previously taken Yoga lessons. With only a small investment, you can gauge your interest in Yoga and see whether you like the instructor. If you don't need much individual attention, if you enjoy doing Yoga together with other people, and if your budget is limited, you will be content with group classes.

On the other hand, you may not like to do Yoga surrounded by others. You may want to progress more quickly than is possible in a group, where those who don't practice at home tend to hold back the rest. You may want to do asanas in unconventional ways and novel juxtapositions, which would be disruptive in a group class. You may want to concentrate only on particular aspects of Yoga, and not have to sit through things that don't interest you.

Moreover, you may want to have the full attention of your teacher. You may want to be able to ask questions freely. You may want to vary the course depending on how you feel that day. You may have a physical condition which holds you back in the group class, but which might respond to adaptations and modifications of the poses designed just for you. If any of these circumstances apply to you, private lessons might be worth trying.

Q: I don't want to draw away from other people. I depend on those around me, and many people depend on me. I believe that such interrelationships are the framework of society. Frankly, I am put off by the self-centered, antisocial image Yoga has. What right have I to indulge in solitary meditative practices, however gratifying personally, when there is so much useful work to be done in the world and so little time to do it in?

A: An eloquent and fundamental objection. Allow me to sidestep it, for the time being, by turning some questions back at you:

- Does the image you have of Yoga derive from personal experience or from the media?

- Is it an indulgence to take minimal preventive care of your body?

- Will a little time spent in getting to know yourself better hamper you in relating to others?

- Is action so pressing that you cannot afford any time for reflection?

- Forgive me; these are intrusive questions. But anyone who would condemn Yoga must, in all fairness, consider them. Meanwhile, let us proceed. The following chapters have been written to clarify what Yoga is and is not, both as a system of physical culture and as an attitude toward life.

3

A MODEL PRACTICE SEQUENCE

And now here is a basic Yoga course, presented in four stages. It is safe, balanced, and complete. Instructions are given here, but explanation of the principles underlying them will be reserved for the next chapter. The course is intended not so much to establish a standardized routine as to illustrate how a series of asanas can be effectively combined for economy and positive results. In Chapter 9, some hints will be given on putting together a Yoga course designed to meet your individual needs. In the meantime, you might experiment with the Model Sequence.

Each stage in the Sequence is designed to be a model course in its own right. Begin with Course #1, and stay with it until you feel the need to incorporate some new material; then go on to Course #2. Proceed by stages at your own pace, keeping in mind that each course will take a little more practice time than the previous one.

In this chapter, the asanas will be referred to by English equivalents of their traditional Sanskrit names. The latter can be found in Chapter 5.

Along with instructions for each of the exercises is line drawings showing the positions between which the movement takes place, and the breathing which accompanies that movement.

- The symbol "Inhale ➤" between two positions means: Inhale as you move from the first position to the second.

- The symbol "Exhale ➤" between two positions means: Exhale as you move from the first position to the second.

- The indication "3 times" means: Perform the movement, with indicated breathing, three times.

- The direction "Stay 1 breath" means: Maintain the indicated posture for one complete breath before resuming the movement.

- The letters R & L represent right and left.

COURSE #1

Course #1 should take you half an hour or less, and consists of six items.

1. Arm-Raise

Begin by standing with feet parallel, either together or slightly spread. Don't lock the legs, but instead keep the knees slightly relaxed. Let the arms hang loosely at your sides, the chin toward the chest. Close your eyes.

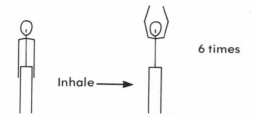

6 times

Inhale ──→

Inhale through the nose, as slowly and evenly as you can. As you inhale, raise the arms gradually from your sides to a position comfortably overhead. Keep the elbows relaxed. When your inhalation is finished, wait for a moment.

Then exhale, also through the nose, simultaneously lowering the arms to their starting position at your sides. Wait a moment. This completes one cycle.

Perform the exercise a total of 6 times (i.e., 6 complete breaths) in succession. Then go on to:

2. Floor-Touch

Inhale, raising the arms overhead.

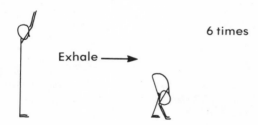

6 times

Exhale ──→

Now, exhaling, bend the trunk forward, letting the legs bend slightly, so that the forehead comes toward the kneecaps, and the fingers come close to the floor. Wait a moment.

On inhalation, return to the starting position. Wait a moment. At the end of the sixth repetition, lower the arms to your sides while exhaling. This completes Floor-Touch. Now proceed to:

3. Triangle Twist

Stand with your feet 2½ to 4 feet apart. Inhaling, extend the arms sideways at shoulder level, palms down.

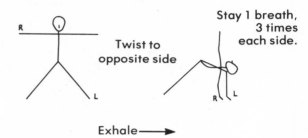

Twist to opposite side

Stay 1 breath, 3 times each side.

Exhale ──→

Exhaling, simultaneously twist and bend down, so that the right hand touches the floor near the left foot. The left leg may bend as much as necessary. The left arm will now be pointing toward the ceiling. The entire spine, starting from the low back, should be gently twisted toward the left. Turn the head so that you are looking at the upraised left hand.

Remain in this position while inhaling and exhaling once. Then, on the second inhalation, come up to the starting position. Wait for a moment.

Now, exhaling, turn and bend toward the right side. Stay one complete breath as before. Then come up inhaling. This makes one full cycle. Repeat to left and right another two times, for a total of three. Lower the arms, exhaling.

4. Quadruped

Instead of two positions, this asana variation has three. They form a reversible sequence; thus, each cycle or set has the order: 1-2-3-2-1.

Kneel on your mat, arms at sides, as if about to pray, toenails touching the mat.

1.   Inhale and raise the arms overhead.

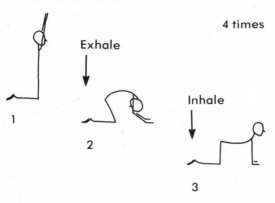

2.   Exhale and bend forward at the hips. Place hands on the mat, about 2 feet in front of the knees. Spread the hands about as far apart as the width of your shoulders. Slightly bend the elbows.

3.   Inhale and glide forward, gradually straightening the arms. Let your back go hollow. Lift the chin.

4.   Exhale and glide backward to Position 2. Try to reverse the curvature of the back, making it as round as possible, from hips to head, like a camel's hump. Let the elbows bend slightly.

5.   Inhaling, lift the arms off the ground and straighten up, still on the knees, into Position 1.

You have now completed one cycle. Do three more. Then lie down on your back.

5.   Supine Rest.

It is important that you rest at this point. Don't try to save time.

Simply lie flat with legs slightly spread, feet turned out, and arms a little away from the body, palms up.

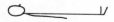

Rest 2 minutes.

Breathe normally and remain still for at least two minutes. Get up only when you are fully rested.

6.   Seated Breathing (Prāṇayāmā)

Seat yourself however you are most comfortable—on a chair, a cushion, or directly on your mat—with your back as straight as possible. Close your eyes, rest your hands, get settled, and breathe quietly (through the nose) for a minute.

Now you are ready to do pranayama.

Breathe in slowly. Wait for a moment. Then begin to let the breath out, making the exhalation last as long as you comfortably can. Wait for a moment, then begin the second breath.

Continue breathing in this manner until you have completed 20 cycles. Then, discontinue the long exhalations, but remain seated in the same position for an additional 2 minutes.

Your Yoga practice is now over. You can return to your normal activities.

Stay with this course for some time, until it is quite familiar to you and well under control. Don't be in a hurry. Only when it is becoming too routinized and no longer requires much attention should you move on to Course #2.

COURSE #2

The Second Course is like the First, with the addition of two asanas between Supine Rest and Seated Breathing.

Items 1-5, by way of review, are:

1.   Arm-Raise

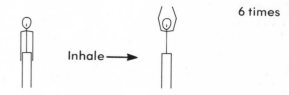

2. Floor-Touch

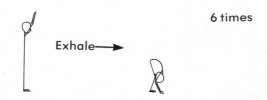

6 times

Exhale →

3. Triangle Twist

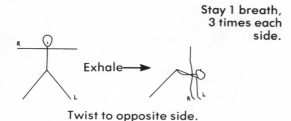

Stay 1 breath,
3 times each
side.

Exhale →

Twist to opposite side.

4. Quadruped

4 times

Exhale →   Inhale →

1   2   3

5. Supine Rest

Rest 2 minutes.

Now add the following:

6. Cobra

Lie prone with arms at your sides and forehead (rather than chin) touching the mat.

Up & down
4 times;
then stay
2 breaths,
2 times.

Inhale →

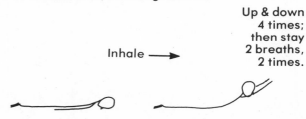

As you inhale, lift the chest and arms off the mat, while at the same time sweeping the arms sideways and forward, with elbows relaxed. Keep the facial muscles and neck relaxed also; it is not important to crane the neck and look at the ceiling.

As you exhale, slowly sweep the arms back to the sides, while lowering the chest and forehead to the mat. Perform this cycle 4 times.

Having inhaled and lifted a fifth time, keep chest and arms above the ground and take 2 full breaths, as slowly as possible. Then, exhaling, return to the starting position. Repeat.

Then roll over onto your back and do:

7. Knee Hold

Lie on the back with legs bent.

Exhale →

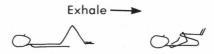

Stay 1 minute.

On exhalation, slowly bring the thighs toward the belly. Hold the knees just below the kneecap. Remain in this position for at least one minute, breathing normally. Then return the feet to the floor and slowly extend the legs.

8. Supine Rest

Rest 1 minute.

Once again rest fully on the back, this time for at least one minute.

9. Seated Breathing

This is identical with Item 6 in Course #1.

COURSE #3

We begin again with the same five asanas (see page 26-27). But at this point we introduce the following:

6. Shoulderstand

Begin by lying on your mat. Be sure there is adequate (but firm and level) padding under your neck and elbows.

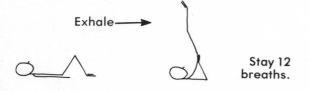

Exhale ➝

Stay 12 breaths.

Exhaling, press the palms against the mat and lift the legs over the head. Then place the palms against the lower back for support, fingers pointing upward.

Remain in Shoulderstand while continuing to breathe slowly and deeply. See if you can gradually work up to 12 breaths. If you like, you may bend the legs with each exhalation, extending them upward on inhalation.

To come out of the pose, bend and lower the legs over the head, exhaling. Lower the arms to the mat. Then, inhaling, slowly roll out onto the mat, keeping legs bent. First the upper back touches, then lower back and feet. Now you can extend the legs along the floor.

7. Supine Rest

Rest 1 minute.

It is important to rest on the back for a little while immediately after Shoulderstand. Then continue, as in Course #2, with:

8. Cobra

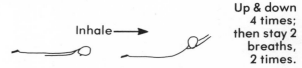

Inhale ➝

Up & down
4 times;
then stay 2
breaths,
2 times.

9. Knee Hold

Stay 1 minute.

10. Supine Rest

Rest 1 minute.

11.   Seated Breathing

Sit and compose yourself as before, and do 20 rounds of long-exhalation breathing. If you like, you may incorporate the following refinement:

Count seconds mentally while inhaling. Wait for a moment. Then exhale, counting, making the exhalation last twice as long as the inhalation. Wait for a moment.

Continue breathing in and out, slowly, in the ratio 1:2. For example, if your inhalation took 3 counts, make the exhalation last for 6. If inhalation is 6 counts, exhalation should be 12. The counts don't have to be seconds exactly, but try to keep them even.

If it becomes a strain to draw out the exhalation, pause and take a few normal breaths, or try reducing slightly the length of inhalation. If 6.12 is too much, drop back to 5.10 and see if it is more manageable. On the other hand, if 3.6 isn't enough of a challenge, you could move up to 4.8.

After completing 20 cycles, discontinue the 1:2 ratio, but remain seated for at least 2 minutes more.

COURSE #4

By appending two more asanas, we shall now complete the Model Sequence. Items 1-10 are as in Course #3:

1. Arm-Raise
2. Floor-Touch
3. Triangle Twist
4. Quadruped
5. Supine Rest
6. Shoulderstand
7. Supine Rest
8. Cobra
9. Knee Hold
10. Supine Rest

Now before going on to Seated Breathing, do the following:

11.   Sitting Stretch

Sit with your legs extended in front of you. Feel free to bend the knees slightly, or to spread the heels apart a few inches.

Inhaling, raise your arms overhead and try to sit up straight.

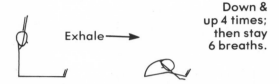

Exhale ——→

Down & up 4 times; then stay 6 breaths.

Exhaling, bend over. Let the hands come to the mat.

Perform this movement 4 times. Then, having bent over again, hold the legs and take 6 deep, slow breaths. Then, on an inhalation, sit up and raise the arms overhead. Lower the arms on exhalation, and proceed to:

12.   Table

Sit with legs extended in front of you. Place your palms on the mat, several inches behind the hips, and about as widely spaced as your shoulders. Fingers should point toward the feet. Bend the knees and place the feet on the floor. Keep the feet apart.

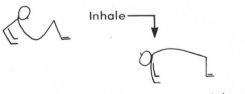

Inhale ——→

4 times

Inhaling, press palms and soles, and lift the hips high off the mat, allowing the head to tip backward.

Exhaling, lower the hips to the mat and the chin to the chest.

Repeat 4 times, then lie down on the back and rest, as indicated in the following two poses:

13. Knee Hold

Stay 1 minute.

14. Supine Rest

Rest 2 minutes

Conclude, as before, with:

15. Seated Breathing.

As in Course #3. Possibly by now you will have noticed an increase in the length of the breath.

Course #4 constitutes the Model Practice Sequence in full. Asanas, pranayama, and resting, all together, will probably take you no more than 45 minutes.

For those interested in a deeper understanding of Yoga practice, Chapter 4 will explain the principles underlying the Model Sequence. Some of these will pertain only to the items selected, but most will be of general application.

4

EXPLAINING THE SEQUENCE

In its final form, as Course #4, the Model Practice Sequence contains eight active asanas with rest intervals, followed by several minutes of seated breathing. Soon we shall examine each of these elements to see why they constitute a model sequence. You may wonder why the Sequence was not introduced in its final form or why it was taken apart and presented piecemeal in four stages.

The explanation is, that although it may be a reasonable objective for most people, Course #4 may not be feasible from the outset for a beginner. Yoga is a progressive endeavor at all levels. Having determined a goal, you assess your present position, and then chart a step-by-step course to take you from here to there. Needless to say, the goal must be realistic and the course appropriate. You have to work within your limitations, even while striving to extend those limitations.

So Yoga involves patience, prudence, and perseverance. Course #1 asks you merely to do some basic stretches, from a standing position and on all fours. After resting, you are asked to si and watch your breath for several minutes, making a slight effort to extend the exhalations. The Course is compact and takes less than half an hour, but you have only to try it to realize that it is thoroughgoing and not at all trivial. Where is the urgency

to go directly to headstands, handstands, or lotuses? These poses may be fine if you have worked up to them; if not, they may do you more harm than good. If you start with Course #1 and practice it for a few weeks, you will have conditioned your body to the point where you can easily cope with the challenge of Course #2.

That challenge, in a word, is Cobra: a classic asana for strengthening the back. If you are comfortable with Course #1, and continue to use it as a warm-up, Cobra should present no great obstacle.

Course #3 introduces Shoulderstand, a valuable asana requiring careful preparation. The course also contains a refinement for Seated Breathing.

Ultimately the Sequence is rounded off, in Course #4, by two complementary seated postures. By this time your Cobra may have become a deep stretch indeed, so a good forward bend is in order. After Sitting Stretch comes Table, to relax the midsection, followed by the usual resting period.

With asanas and pranayama practiced step by step in this way, body and mind have a chance to adapt themselves without pain, strain, or frustration. If, however, you still find parts of the Model Sequence too difficult, you might consult Chapter 5, which illustrates a variety of basic āsanas, some of which may be more practicable; and Chapter 9, which indicates how you can tailor your Yoga course to your individual requirements. If the Model Sequence is too easy for you, you should at least have an inkling of how you might intensify it.

MOVEMENT IN ASANAS

Judging from the Model Practice Sequence, you would have to conclude that movement is an essential component of asana. Yet many books on Yoga show a single, motionless position for each asana. And, as we have noted, the word *āsana* literally means "posture." How shall we account for this discrepancy?

First of all, we must concede that it is impossible to be truly motionless unless one holds one's breath the whole time. As long as one is breathing, there will always be some movement in the trunk, even if the limbs are relatively immobile. And, as we shall see, the effect of an asana is heightened, not diminished, by breathing. So the issue is not so much "movement versus non-movement," as "maximum movement versus minimum movement." Which is the more desirable?

Whether you do an asana dynamically or statically depends on your physical condition and your purpose in choosing the asana. Doing an asana dynamically takes the body through a larger arc of movement. Thus, more muscle groups are called into play, and there is more skeletal activity around the joints. Since the lungs have a chance to expand fully and deflate completely, there is inducement to deeper breathing. Repeated movements are effective as warm-ups, and as compensatory stretches after asanas which make intense demands on the opposite sets of muscles. Doing asanas dynamically is also the best preparation for doing them statically. Instances of all these uses are found in the Model Practice Sequence, and will be commented on individually.

By contrast, static performance of asanas eliminates obvious movement, and presupposes considerable flexibility. There is relatively little activity at the joints, no rhythmical muscular contractions, and less encouragement to complete respiration. Clearly, static asanas are not suited for use as warm-ups or counterposes.

But there is a positive side. By minimizing limb movement you can work more on stretching the vertebrae and on developing your staying power. Held postures might appear to exercise fewer muscle groups, but as superficial muscles begin to tire, deeper ones are innervated. These are often poorly developed, and scarcely come into play during dynamic stretching. And the longer the pose is held, the more you will feel sympathetic contractions spreading throughout the body. To be sure, not all static poses increase muscular effort; some are simply more restful.

Compared to their dynamic variations, static asanas have a more internal effect; they provide an opportunity to feel things happening deep within. Certainly, you cannot claim to have mastered an asana before you can remain in it comfortably with controlled breathing. In theory, asana is indeed motionless; but for it eventually to be so, with comfort equal to effort, it must begin as liberal movement.

SLOW MOTION

All movement in asana should be slow. Among the advantages of slow motion are:

1. Heightened attention. Most of us are unused to moving our body parts in a smooth, graceful manner. Movements in daily life are usually unmeasured and unpremeditated. Movements in other forms of exercise may be rhythmical, but tend to be rapid or automatic. The very novelty and unfamiliarity of slow Yoga movements demand considerable mental attention. "Attention in action" is one of the defining characteristics of Yoga.

2. Decreased risk of muscle strain or joint injury. When muscles are made to contract violently and repeatedly, they are easily strained, along with the ligaments surrounding the joints. Delicate joint structures may be affected. You may be oblivious to strain or injury until long after. Exercising slowly with attention, you can be sensitive to the first signals of strain, and can stop well before any damage is done.

3. Involvement of more muscles. In rapid movement, the work is done by the muscles that are strongest. In slow movement, other muscle groups are called upon to participate, sharing the work more evenly.

4. Quicker relaxation. Muscles relax on being stretched by the contraction of opposing muscles, and when the chemical by-products of contraction are removed by the blood. Slow movement permits deeper stretching of tight muscles. At the same time, it encourages more thorough removal of by-products (lactic acid, carbon dioxide, etc,), and more ample supply of oxygen and glucose to fuel subsequent contractions.

5. Improved circulation. Slow movement puts no sudden strain on the heart, but does encourage it to pump more regularly and forcefully. Since more muscle groups are contracting more efficiently, the work load of the heart is eased and circulation is improved. Exercising slowly and with attention, you can easily stop before overtaxing the heart.

6. Improve respiration. When you exercise slowly, your muscles won't build up an oxygen debt and you won't get out of breath. Deep, controlled breathing during exercise increases the capacity and elasticity of the lungs, and the efficiency of the entire respiratory system.

COORDINATING MOVEMENT AND BREATH

For maximum effectiveness, all asana movements should be accompanied by conscious breathing. Instructions on when to breathe in and out have been given for each of the asanas in the Model Sequence, based on two simple principles:

1. *Inhale* when executing a movement which naturally encourages the *expansion* of the lungs.

2. *Exhale* when the movement encourages *deflation* of the lungs.

The movement corresponding to inhalation should normally have the same rate of speed as the movement corresponding to exhalation. In other words, breathing in and breathing out should be adjusted to take roughly the same amount of time.

An often repeated instruction in the Model Practice Sequence is to "wait for a moment" in between the phases of the breath—that is, before exhalation and again before inhalation. This interval is not tantamount to holding the breath; it need not last more than one or two seconds. Its function is merely to articulate, or punctuate, the two phases of the breath/movement cycle. Yoga movements should not be circular or completely continuous, lest breathing become uneven and attention wane.

In Yoga it is always desirable to breathe through the nose. The mouth is not as well designed for respiration. Use your mouth if you have to, but make an effort to develop the habit of nose breathing. See Chapter 6 for further discussion of this and other matters relating to breath.

A WORD ON EFFECTS

Writers on Yoga have always been tempted to ascribe specific "effects" or "benefits" to asanas and pranayama. It would indeed be convenient if the mechanics and therapeutic range of every asana could be scientifically established. But it is obvious that people will react differently to an asana, depending on their age, constitution, background in Yoga, and the manner in which they use the asana. For that matter, the same person will react differently to the same asana, given a change of physical condition, state of mind, time of day, etc.

How then can we predict categorically the effect that an asana will have on an organ or system? An asana encouraging a healthy muscular development in one person may aggravate another's delicate joints. An asana designed to take care of one problem may inadvertently cause others. A difficult or dangerous posture may be attempted in order to obtain a desired result, when a simpler or safer one would do the job. Since there are so many variables involved, we shall try not to make undemonstrable claims for the asanas and pranayama under consideration.

Returning to the Model Practice Sequence, let us look at each of its components.

Arm-Raise

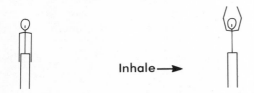

Inhale →

The first priority of any exercise session is to get more blood to the muscles and joints. The extremities tend to be stiffer and colder than the trunk, especially after sleep. Simple bending and stretching movements done slowly will deepen your breathing and stimulate circulation.

In principle, warm-up stretches are best done from a standing position. Lying on the back may be too restful, while sitting may not permit enough movement (though persons who have difficulty standing may find these positions quite useful for doing mild exercise). Standing offers no impediment to deep breathing and permits a wide range of invigorating movement.

Lifting and lowering the arms is a convenient way to start. Raising the arms promotes fuller ventilation of the lungs, by stretching the spine, and mechanically assisting the lifting of the upper ribs. As the upper ribs lift, the lower ribs tend to spread out, and the lungs are expanded. Conversely, lowering the arms helps retract the ribs, favoring exhalation.

In keeping with its role as a warm-up, Arm-Raise is to be performed dynamically. It should be repeated enough times to produce the desired effect without causing fatigue. Six repetitions are suggested, but you may find that four are sufficient; or you may need eight to get any effect out of the exercise. Adjust accordingly. As a rule, it is better to do fewer repetitions with deep breathing than many repetitions with rapid breathing.

Apart from extending the breath, Arm-Raise helps to loosen the shoulder joints. Since these are often stiff, you are cautioned to "raise the arms gradually...to a position comfortably overhead. Keep the elbows relaxed." Don't try to stretch your arms beyond the point at which you first feel resistance.

Like other standing asanas, Arm-Raise draws attention to and helps correct poor postural habits. Avoid locking the legs, but try instead to keep the knees slightly relaxed. You may spread the feet for greater stability, though later on you can practice the asana with feet parallel and close together.

The instructions ask you to close your eyes, since visual stimuli may draw attention from your movements and breathing. If, however, you feel unsteady or disoriented, you should leave the eyes open.

Floor-Touch

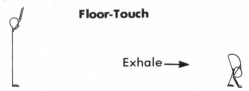

Exhale →

Floor-Touch is also an excellent warm-up, but is more intense than Arm-Raise. There is no change in the stance, and the position on completion of inhalation is identical to Arm-Raise. On exhalation, however, you lower not just the arms but the entire trunk. Chest and abdomen being squeezed, it obviously makes sense to exhale.

It is important to differentiate Floor-Touch, as a Yoga asana, from the calisthenic exercise that, on paper, resembles it. Floor-Touch is to be performed as *slowly* as your breath allows; six repetitions will do. The object here is not to lock the legs and "bounce" the trunk, until the fingers reach the toes. On the contrary, you should bend the legs freely, so that the fingers (ultimately the entire palm) can touch the floor.

Bending over with legs locked can strain the leg and low-back muscles. Instead of loosening the stiffer parts of the spine, you may be overstretching the looser areas. Rather than improving your posture, you may be endangering a frail low back or exaggerating a round upper back. You could also strain the neck or shoulders.

Relaxing the legs allows you to put a controlled stretch on the big flexor muscles of the leg (the hamstrings), which in many people are very tight. It also increases mobility in the low back—another typically stiff area. Hip joints, too, are progressively loosened. The stretching effect can be felt all along the spinal column, right up to the neck.

Move the chin toward the throat, as far as is comfortable. Keep elbows and shoulders relaxed.

Floor-Touch is a marvelous exercise for developing correct breathing habits. The flexed position encourages complete emptying of the lungs, while the erect position favors complete expansion. Rationing the inflow and outflow of air through almost 180 degrees of slow motion is a good test for breath control.

The practice of Floor-Touch will accustom you to the head-below-heart position. Besides mildly stimulating blood flow to the neck, the bent-over position prepares you gradually for more dramatic, fully inverted postures to come.

Arm-Raise and Floor-Touch can be used to advantage, not only at the beginning of a Yoga practice, but as a conditioning warm-up for sports and other physical activities.

Triangle Twist

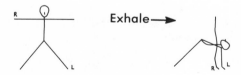

Exhale →

Arm-Raise and Floor-Touch are good exercises for extension and flexion of the trunk. In the course of our normal activities we all bend and straighten our backs to some extent. Less often we make use of the third basic type of movement possible for the vertebral column—rotation. Triangle Twist is therefore a particularly valuable exercise.

The instructions ask you to spread your feet apart by 2½ to 4 feet. The proper width depends on your height and the elasticity of your leg muscles. The spread-leg stance allows you to stretch not only the hamstring and calf muscles, but those along the inside of the thigh (adductors). You may also notice some tightness around the hips, since spreading the legs restricts mobility at the joints.

You are told, as you inhale, to extend the arms sideways at shoulder level, palms down. (Turning palms up may cause pain in the shoulder region.) Exhaling, place your right hand near the left foot—on the instep side to start with, but on the outside when you become more expert. You may bend the left leg as much as necessary. Here again, as in Floor-Touch, bending the leg permits greater mobility in the vertebral column.

Each vertebra can only move a little further than the one beneath it, but the combined effect is significant. Flexion and extension occur in the way one might build an arch out of bricks or stones, while the mechanism of rotation is analogous to a spiral staircase. The Latin word *vertebra*, in fact, means "something to turn on."

Try to feel that you are twisting as mucn as possible from the back. Otherwise you may compensate by overtwisting the neck. Having then turned the trunk and shoulders, turn the head gently, so that you are looking at the upraised left hand.

Triangle Twist, alone among the asanas in the Model Sequence, illustrates the use of asymmetrical poses. No human body ever develops truly symmetrically; there will always be minor disparities between left and right. It is when these are reinforced and magnified by habit or laziness that serious problems may arise. Long, strong muscles run up the legs, along each side of the spine, and down the arms. If one member or one side becomes weak through disuse or injury, the body will favor it and make the other side work a little harder.

Unchecked, the weak muscles tend to become weaker and the strong muscles stronger. Similarly, joints that are not exercised will lose flexibility. To insure that both sides of the body are being developed equally, you should include side-stretching and twisting movements in your exercise program. Asymmetrical poses will tell you a great deal about your body structure and eccentricities of posture.

Like most Yoga postures, Triangle Twist works deeply on the low back and abdomen. This central region of the body, so vital to health, is all too often neglected. Stiffness in the lumbar spine, and the weak musculature which usually accompanies it, are at the root of many back troubles, and result in postural fatigue. When there are problems in the back, it is not a coincidence that there are usually problems in front as well. The abdomen contains all the important viscera except the heart and lungs. It is the home of the digestive and genital organs. A stiff back means an under-exercised abdomen. Poor muscle tone in the abdominal wall leads to fatty accumulation and offers insufficient support to the viscera. These get squeezed out of proper alignment and begin to press upon one another, causing various obstructions and dysfunctions. Asanas with breathing provide an excellent abdominal massage, particularly twists.

Since rotation compresses the chest and abdomen, for best effect you should exhale while twisting. Inhale as you come back to the starting position. In Triangle Twist we have introduced a new technicality: after twisting to the left side, you are told to "remain in this position while inhaling and exhaling once." In strenuous asanas involving deep stretching, it is often advisable to pause for a breath in between movements. While catching your breath, you are at the same time benefiting from holding the pose a little longer. Then when you resume the movement you will have breath enough to keep it slow and controlled. Since you are holding the pose for a breath each time, three repetitions per side should suffice.

In order to realign the muscles and joints, you should always follow a twisting asana with a forward bend. Having just done a standing twist you could do a standing bend, but as your legs may be tired after three successive standing asanas, you may find it relaxing to get off your feet while you do the counterpose. Accordingly, the Model Practice Sequence continues with a series of stretches done on the knees.

Quadruped

Exhale

Inhale

We have taken some liberty in rendering *Chakravākāsana* as "Quadruped." *Chakravāka*

is actually a mythical bird, akin to a goose. However, Chakravākāsana admits of many variations, some of which may not resemble a bird at all. Quadruped, in a simpler form, is illustrated in Chapter 5. The version we are using here, as a counterpose to Triangle Twist, has you kneel to start. It has three positions instead of the usual two. Each set entails two full breaths, so four repetitions should be adequate.

Kneeling postures exercise the knee joints, stretch the thighs, and require bracing action in the calf, hamstring, and buttocks muscles. In Kneeling—unlike standing—postures, you can bend deeply even if your legs are stiff. If you are unaccustomed to kneeling you may appreciate a pillow or soft pad placed under the knees.

From the starting position with arms raised, exhale and bend forward. Place your hands on the mat, about two feet in front of the knees to have a stable base for gliding forward and back. The knees should be spread about as far apart as the width of your shoulders and your elbows should be slightly bent. In this way the joints are protected and the muscles do the work.

Inhale and glide forward, gradually straightening the arms. Let your back go hollow. Lift the chin. With the weight of the trunk shared by arms and thighs, you can fully and comfortably extend the entire vertebral column. Then, as you exhale, glide backward to Position 2. Try to reverse the curvature of the back, making it as round as possible, from hips to head, like a camel's hump. Just as you can conveniently hollow the back on all fours, so can you nicely stretch it the other way as well. This phase of the asana is particularly relaxing to the low back and neck. Let the chin move toward the chest as far as it wants to. Once again bend the elbows. Resume Position 1 on inhalation.

Supine Rest

Shoulderstand

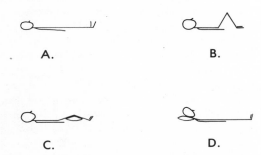

A.

B.

C.

D.

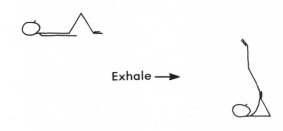

Exhale ⟶

After Quadruped, you are asked to lie down on your back. It's a good idea even if you don't think you need to.

Simply lie flat with legs slightly spread, feet turned out, and arms a little away from the body, palms up as shown in Fig. A. These instructions could be condensed to one word: Relax!—but that is easier said than done. Lying as described puts you in the most favorable attitude for relaxation. If you suffer from back pain you may feel more comfortable resting with legs bent (Fig. B), or with a cushion under the knees (Fig. C). If your neck is stiff, place a pillow under your head (Fig. D). Let the breath come naturally. You need not employ any techniques of auto-suggestion; having exercised well you will relax well.

Taking a brief rest several times during your practice keeps you from getting exhausted and improves your endurance. Resting lets the mind catch up with the body and register the effects of the previous asana. Never hesitate to lie down for a while at any point in your practice, even where not indicated in the instructions.

Sarvāṅgāsana literally means "All-Parts-" or "Entire-Body-Pose," but it is commonly translated as "Shoulderstand."

The instructions ask you to be sure there is adequate (but firm and level) padding under neck and elbows. Extra padding is needed since the elbows, shoulders, and cervical vertebrae are not naturally cushioned for weight-bearing. However, the pad shouldn't be too spongy, or you will be unable to press the elbows firmly and will feel too much pressure in the head.

Exhaling, press the palms against the mat and lift the legs over the head. You may find it easier to bend the knees somewhat before lifting the legs. Then place the palms against the lower back for support, fingers pointing upward. With the hands flat against the back there is minimum pressure on the wrists and elbows and more utilization of the back muscles.

Although you are using your hands to support the back, you should resist the urge to push against it. There is absolutely no need to force the body into a vertical alignment. Your back and neck will stretch as much as they are prepared to, and with practice you will probably notice your legs moving gradually closer to the perpendicular. But if you insist on being as straight as a candlestick (as the pose is sometimes called, unfortunately) you are inviting injury to your neck and upper back. Remember that it has taken years to "develop" your stiff joints and weak muscles; don't begrudge the weeks or months it may take to restore suppleness and strength. For many people even the simplest Shoulderstand is out of the question. If this seems to be the case for you, accept your limitation, and work on simpler asanas for the time being.

You may find it hard to control your breath in Shoulderstand. Do the best you can; deep breathing improves the effect of the pose. Stay for 12 breaths if you can, but by all means come down if you start to tremble or pant. If staying 12 breaths gets to be too easy, first try lengthening the breaths; later you can increase the *number* of breaths—to 16, for example. If you need help in equalizing inhalation and exhalation, or if you find the static pose too taxing, or if you simply get restless, you may bend the legs with each exhalation, extending them upward on inhalation.

Upside-down postures are highly valued in Yoga. They compensate for all the time we spend right-side up. Man has become quite adapted to going about erect on two legs, but if he becomes careless with his body, he soon realizes that his vertebral column was not designed to support ribs and skull, but to *be* supported by four sturdy legs. Unlike other vertebrates, man carries his brain well above his heart; yet his highly developed brain needs a copious blood supply. The circulatory and muscular strain of upright carriage catch up with him periodically, and man must lie down and rest.

It is frequently desirable to lie with the legs elevated above heart and head; hospital beds are engineered to do this for the infirm. For healthy persons, a few minutes spent in Shoulderstand lets the body recuperate from the ill effects of prolonged sitting, standing, or walking.

What happens in Shoulderstand? First of all, blood which has pooled in the legs drains toward the heart. Swelling in the veins is reduced; afterward, the legs should feel lighter, springier. Muscles in the abdomen and back contract to support the weight of the legs, while the entire vertebral column is stretched, particularly in the neck. The increased blood flow to the neck is thought, among other things, to benefit the thyroid gland, whose healthy functioning is important for proper metabolism.

If Shoulderstand makes you feel better, you will have motivation enough to do it often. But if it makes you feel worse—and you are sure you are following the instructions—then obviously it isn't for you just yet.

If you practice Headstand or are interested in learning it, you will find Shoulderstand especially useful. Chapters 7 and 9 explain why. If you want to practice Shoulderstand apart from the Model Sequence, you should prepare for it by doing some asanas and then resting on the back.

To come down from Shoulderstand, bend and lower the legs over the head, as you exhale. Lower the arms to the mat. Then, as you inhale, slowly roll out onto the mat, keeping legs bent. First uncurl the back, then let your feet touch down. The spinal column has been bearing the considerable weight of pelvis and legs, and need to be eased to the ground gradually. After you have stretched out the legs along the floor, it is important that you remain in that restful position for a minute or more. The longer your Shoulderstand, the longer you should rest. Ribs and vertebrae need time to readjust, muscles to relax, and circulation to normalize.

Cobra

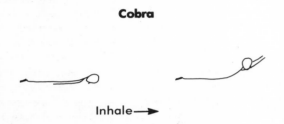

Inhale ➝

The next asana in the Model Practice Sequence is Cobra. The instructions direct you to lie prone with arms at your sides and forehead (rather than chin) touching the mat. As you inhale, lift the chest and arms off the mat, at the same time sweeping the arms sideways and forward, with elbows relaxed. Lifting the arms insures that you will use Cobra not as a push-up but as a "pull-up"; after all, a real cobra lifts its head without benefit of limbs. Sweeping the arms shifts forward the body's center of gravity, and distributes the work of lifting more evenly through the back. It also loosens up the neck, shoulders, and elbows— which were immobilized and weight-bearing in Shoulderstand.

Keep the facial muscles and neck relaxed also; it is not important to crane the neck and look at the ceiling. The purpose of Cobra is to extend the entire vertebral column—not primarily the neck, which is already predisposed to curve backward. Tensing the facial muscles indicates you are working too hard from the neck up.

As you exhale, slowly sweep the arms back to the sides, while lowering the chest and forehead

to the mat. Perform this cycle 4 times. Now you can stay longer in the posture. Inhaling and lifting yet again, keep chest and arms above the ground and take 2 full breaths, as slowly as possible. Then, exhaling, return to the starting position. Repeat. Staying in Cobra for a few breaths at a time requires the back to work even harder, and is effective if you have first prepared the back muscles to develop strength by dynamic repetitions.

In Shoulderstand, the back is rounded under the weight of the legs, and the abdomen is in forced contraction. Cobra has the opposite effect: the back is extended, against gravity, and the abdomen is stretched. So the asanas are complementary. Cobra is certainly worth trying even if you don't feel ready for Shoulderstand, but you may have to reduce the number of repetitions and eliminate the static phase.

Cobra, too, needs a counterpose, if only briefly. The best one is:

Knee Hold

Stay 1 minute.

Knee Hold is a most versatile relaxing pose. Ideal after Cobra, it is advisable after any asana involving extension of the back or stretching of the legs. It stretches the back and relaxes the legs, while you rest and resume normal breathing. If you feel tense around the neck, rest your head on a pillow. Knee Hold may also be used apart from your regular Yoga practice. It is helpful at times of bellyache, constipation, and back pain.

A minute or more of Supine Rest completes the relaxation process.

Sitting Stretch

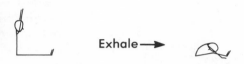

Exhale ➤

In structuring the Model Practice Sequence, we used a group of standing and kneeling stretches to build up to Shoulderstand and Cobra. Now comes the tapering-off phase, which is basically about sitting: a seated asana with its counterpose, a final rest period, and several minutes of Seated Breathing.

Sitting Stretch, like Floor-Touch, looks like a well-known calisthenic; but as in Floor-Touch, the object is not to lock the legs and bob up and down rapidly. To get the best stretching effect you must move slowly—with deep, synchronized breathing. You will probably want to keep your legs slightly bent. As you inhale, raise your arms overhead and try to sit up straight. Exhaling, bend over. Let the hands come to the mat. Perform this movement 4 times.

When you sit on the floor with legs extended—and to some extent when you sit on a chair—the pelvis is fixed at an angle which makes the back excessively round. Unless you resist actively, you tend to slump. Slumping sets up tension in the back and neck. It compresses the rib cage and re-

stricts lung expansion. If you will make an exercise out of sitting straight, it helps to strengthen the back muscles and improves posture generally.

Just as raising the arms overhead encourages extension of the vertebrae and deepens inhalation, bending the trunk forward stretches the back and makes exhalation more complete. As in Floor-Touch, allowing the legs to bend may increase the participation of the lower back. It also helps to get at tight hamstring muscles. Sitting Stretch, done dynamically, reduces stiffness in the hip joints and rhythmically massages the organs of the abdomen.

As in Cobra, the dynamic phase precedes and prepares for the static. After four breaths down and up, bend over again, grasp the legs, and stay for six complete breaths. Holding the pose lets you experience the full stretching effect. When you are finished, sit up and do the following counterpose:

Table

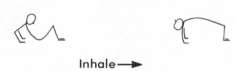

Inhale ➤

Starting from the same seated posture, place your palms on the mat, several inches behind the hips, and about as widely spaced as your shoulders. This positioning helps to transmit weight through the arms to the floor. The fingers should point toward the feet to minimize strain on shoulders and wrists. Bend the knees and place the feet on the floor. Position the feet so that when you lift up, the arms and calves are perpendicular to the floor, like the legs of a table. Keep the feet apart to avoid straining the low back.

Inhaling, press down with palms and soles and lift the hips high off the mat, allowing the head to tip backward. This movement mildly extends the spinal column and stretches the arms, thighs, and abdomen. As you exhale, lower the hips to the mat and the chin to the chest. The Table pose is best done dynamically. If the head were kept dangling, its weight might strain the neck. Lowering hips to mat on each exhalation helps build strength in the arms.

Repeat 4 times, then lie down on the back and rest in Knee Hold position for at least one minute, followed by Supine Rest for at least two. Don't get up until you feel completely rested and your breathing has returned to normal.

Seated Breathing

A classic pose for pranayama is *Siddhāsana*, in which you sit with legs turned outward and folded back inward: one heel at the perineum with the other heel atop it. This posture is illustrated in Chapter 8. You may also sit in some other cross-legged pose, or on your heels, kneeling. Conceivably you may never be at ease in any of these—but that is no reason not to do pranayama. You will just have to sit in less exotic fashion. If you can manage to sit cross-legged, try placing a cushion beneath you, or sit with your back against a wall. If not, sit on a chair. How you sit is secondary, so long as you can hold your back relatively straight. If even sitting on a chair is tiring for you—as it is for everyone at times—do your pranayama lying supine on the mat.

It is best not to begin abruptly. Sit or lie quietly until you are calm and settled. Make no effort to restrain your thoughts. Close your eyes. Be sure you are not inadvertently breathing through the mouth. Only when you feel ready should you begin to control your breathing.

There are many types and techniques of pranayama. The one selected to complete the Model Practice Sequence is known as "long-exhalation," or *rechaka*, pranayama. It is probably the simplest and most relaxing. In Course #1, breathing was unmeasured. Course #3 invited you to begin counting the length of your in- and out-breaths, finding, by trial and error, the maximum length of inhalation that allows you to sustain the exhalation for exactly twice as long. Everyone has a different breath capacity, but anyone can breathe in the ratio 1:2. The instructions explained how to adjust inhalation and exhalation to achieve this ratio.

Note that you are not asked to *hold* the breath, although you are told to suspend the breath for an articulatory movement between the phases—as you have been doing in your asana practice. Pranayama should never be a strain; you may interrupt the breathing pattern and take a few normal breaths whenever you like.

Twenty cycles of conscious long-exhalation breathing should do, but remain seated in the same position for an additional 2 minutes to permit your breathing, heart rate, and mental activity gradually, and gently, to return to normal.

So ends the Model Practice Sequence. We have tried to show why it is safe, balanced, and complete. This is not to say that another sequence would not be. The Model Sequence is but one of an infinite number which could be created in conformity with the same basic principles. It has been our aim to communicate those principles, and not

so much to insist on a specific routine. This particular routine may not suit you. Even if you like it, you
will soon feel the need of some variety. In either
case, you will find useful variations suggested in
the next chapter.

5

AN ANTHOLOGY OF ASANAS

You have seen something of the logic of Yoga. To appreciate also its versatility requires more familiarity with the basic resource of Yoga practice: asanas. Here, with photographs and instructions, is a representative selection. These asanas do not constitute a "course" in any sense, and are not meant to be practiced in consecutive order. For convenience of description we have grouped them into the following classes: supine, standing, all-fours, sitting, prone, and inverted.

This collection of asanas is by no means exhaustive. Think of it rather as a sampler. Many equally important asanas had to be excluded for reasons of space. Fortunately there are already numerous books on Yoga containing complete inventories of the asanas practiced in their respective traditions. We have chosen to illustrate these particular asanas only because:

1. They are relatively safe.
2. The exercise they provide is basic rather than extreme.
3. They present a wide spectrum of movements and postures.
4. Each of them offers considerable scope for variation and adaptation.

5. They embody the principles set forth in this book.
6. Some of them will be referred to in subsequent chapters.
7. Many of them are not found in other books on Yoga.

You will recognize the asanas of the Model Practice Sequence among them. For some of these, additional variations are suggested. If you have been practicing the Model Sequence you will already have a good idea how to use the new asanas, whether by interpolation or substitution. There is little harm in trying to do so. But if you have not practiced the Model Sequence and studied Chapter 4 you should not attempt the asanas in this chapter. Only as you read further will it become clear how to use them to best advantage. Your teacher should be able to explain any discrepancies between the asanas as described here and the way you may have learned them. This book is intended to supplement—not supplant—a teacher.

As in Chapter 3, the asanas will be identified by English names—sometimes unconventional ones. Since there is no standardized nomenclature in English, the original Sanskrit is also given in parentheses. The text of this chapter need not be read through in sequence, but may be dipped into as occasion and curiosity warrant.

Be assured that the persons photographed are neither forcing nor faking. They are doing the poses in a way that is meaningful for them. There is no reason why your renditions must look like theirs. An asana can be represented objectively by a line drawing but it is essentially impossible to photograph. What appears in a photo is no longer an idea but a living person creatively adapting that idea to his or her needs and capacities. Try to emulate not so much the form you see as the effort you can infer.

For most of the asanas two positions are indicated, along with the breathing which accompanies the oscillation between them. You will often be invited to "stay for several breaths" in one or both of these positions. In this way you can experience the motionless quality of asana. Where an asana contains more than two distinct positions, the text explains how to connect them.

Where the version or versions we have given depart significantly from the classic final pose, we have included a photo of the latter. The final pose is not necessarily more advantageous than the preliminary stages, nor is it always more difficult. But it is the symbol of the asana and should be kept in mind.

Wherever there is even a small risk of unwanted side-effects we have suggested one or more counterposes. Which of them works best will depend on you and the effect on you of the asana in question. The crucial role of the counterpose was noted in the previous chapter and will be elaborated on in Chapter 9.

SUPINE ASANAS

Lying on the back is obviously the most restful position in which to exercise. The category of supine asanas features several valuable counterposes, and offers relatively easy access to Yoga for many persons whose physical condition precludes more strenuous postures. The seven asanas we have selected show how you can work on virtually every part of the body while lying on your back. You can also do a great deal with your breath, since the chest is free to expand.

1. SUPINE ARM-RAISE (Supta Tādāsana)

Start from Supine Rest (discussed on page 37).

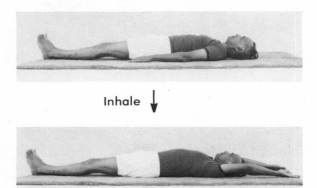

Inhale ↓

Inhaling, lift the arms and move them slowly through 180 degrees, until they come to rest on the mat.

Exhaling, lift them and bring them back to your sides. You may pause for extra breaths with arms in either position.

2. KNEE HOLD (*Apanasana*)

Knee Hold was introduced in the Model Practice Sequence, where it functioned as a resting pose. See page 27 for instructions and page 40 for commentary. If you like, you may incorporate conscious breathing and a small amount of movement, as the photos show.

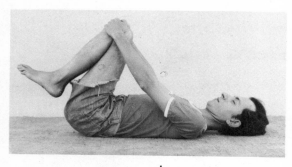

Exhale ↓

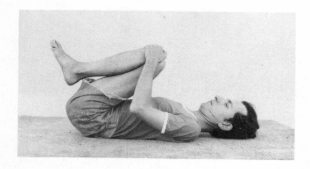

On exhalation, the thighs descend toward the abdomen and the elbows bend.

On inhalation, the arms straighten and the thighs move away from the abdomen.

Suggested counterpose: Supine Rest.

3. LEG LIFT (*Ūrdhava Prasṛta Pādāsana*)

Lie with legs as in Knee Hold, but with arms at sides.

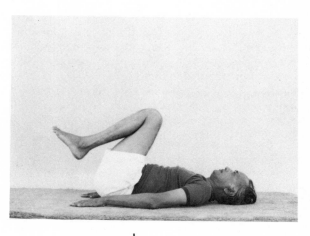

Inhale ↓

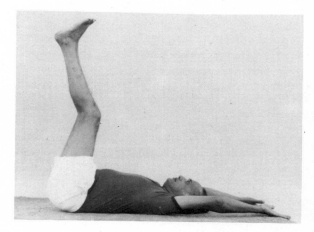

Inhaling, extend the legs upward. It is not necessary that the legs be completely straight or fully vertical. You can enhance the effect of the pose by simultaneously lifting the arms and moving them toward the floor behind your head (as in Supine Arm-Raise).

Exhaling, bend the legs and bring the arms back to the sides.

Having done the asana dynamically, you may want to remain in either position for one or more breaths at a time.

Suggested counterpose: Knee Hold.

4. BRIDGE (*Dvi-Pāda Pīṭha*)

Lie with legs bent and feet on the floor, a comfortable distance apart.

Version 1:

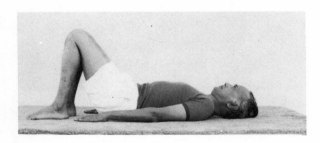

Inhale ↓

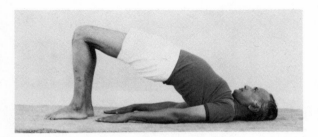

Inhaling, lift the hips and back off the mat.
Exhaling, lower the back gradually to the mat.

Repeat several times; then, if you wish, stay in Bridge for a few additional breaths.

Version 2:

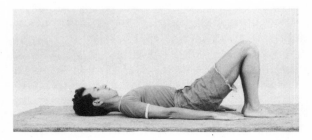

Inhale ↓

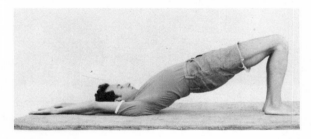

Version 2 adds arm movement as in Supine Arm-Raise and Leg Lift. This position too may be held for several breaths.

In the final pose (not recommended for beginners) the legs are together and the ankles are held.

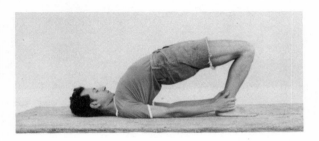

Suggested counterpose: Knee Hold.

5. SUPINE SIDE STRETCH (*Supta Pārshwa Tādāsana*)

Lie on your back with arms at sides. Spread the arms on the mat at shoulder level, palms up. Then inch the legs one by one toward one side until you begin to feel a stretch on the opposite side of the body. The feet should touch each other, with both heels on the floor. Keep the legs in this position.

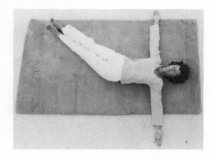

Exhale ↓

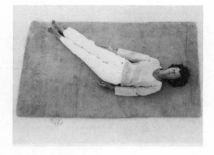

Exhaling, slowly slide the arms back along the floor to your sides.

Inhaling, slide the arms again to the spread position.

Repeat this arm movement several times. Feel free to pause for several breaths in either position. Then, with arms spread, return the legs to the center.

Now move the legs to the other side, sweeping the arms and breathing as before. *Suggested counterpose:* Knee Hold.

6. SUPINE TWIST (*Jathara Parivrtti*)

Lie on your back with arms about 45 degrees away from your sides, palms up. Bend the legs and place the feet on the floor, spread symmetrically apart about 12 inches.

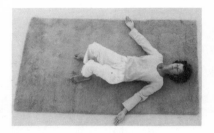

Exhale ↓

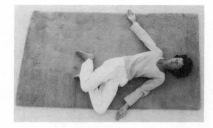

Exhaling, roll the legs toward the floor on one side.

Inhaling, roll back to first Position.

Exhaling, roll to the other side; inhaling, return to first Position.

48

Repeat this cycle several times.

Clearly there are many stages between this simplification and the final pose, shown below, wherein both legs are stretched to one side, toes held by one hand, while the head is turned to the opposite side.

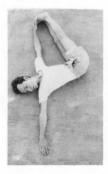

Suggested counterpose: Knee Hold.

7. ONE-LEG SUPINE TWIST (*Eka-Pāda Jathara Parivrtti*)

Lie on your back. Rest your arms on the mat, spread sideways at shoulder level, palms up. Bend one leg—let us say the right—and place its foot on the mat alongside the left leg.

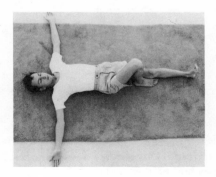

Exhale ↓

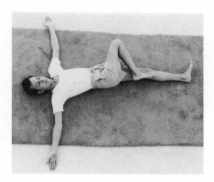

Exhaling, roll the right leg toward the floor on the left side. The right foot may come off the mat, but it should remain pressed against the left leg.

Inhaling, roll back to Position 1.

Repeat several times. You may then stay an additional few breaths in Position 2.

Inhaling, return to Position 1. Stretch out the right leg and bend the left.

Rolling now to the right side, do the asana in the same way for the same number of breaths.

The arm positions we have suggested for this and the preceding two asanas are interchangeable: the arms may be spread at 45 or 90 degrees, depending on the condition of your shoulders; or the arms may be swept out and in with the breath, as in Supine Side Stretch.

In the final position of One-Leg Supine Twist, one leg is stretched to the side and held by the hand. This position is included only for reference; several intermediate steps are necessary before it can be achieved.

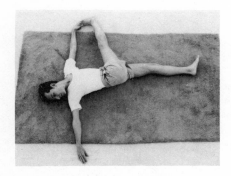

Suggested counterpose: Knee Hold.

STANDING ASANAS

Standing asanas are useful for warming up, for stretching and strengthening the back and the legs, and for improving the balancing faculty. For these reasons they are excellent preludes to all upright activities. Their value in Yoga is augmented by their action in deepening respiration. We have selected eleven standing asanas as representative.

8. ARM-RAISE (*Sama-Sthiti*)

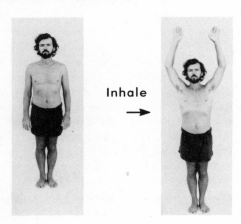

Inhale →

Arm-Raise was the first asana in the Model Practice Sequence. See page 24 for instructions and pages 34-35 for commentary. Although it is not evident from the photos, the arms may be raised to the sides as well as to the front of the body.

Having several times raised and lowered the arms in conjunction with slow in-and-out breathing, you can remain in the arms-raised position for an additional few breaths. Or, alternatively, you can pause for one or more breaths in between the up and down movements of the arms. Or you can pause for a breath in the middle of the movement, holding the arms at the halfway point. Such variations are optional, but come in handy when you want to liven up postures that have become stale through repeated practice.

9. PALM TREE (*Tādāsana*)

This is Arm-Raise with a difference.

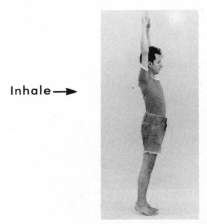

Inhale →

The arm movement and breathing are familiar, but on inhalation you elevate the heels and balance on the toes and metatarsals.

The heels return to the floor as you exhale.

As you become proficient in Palm Tree you will be able to remain with heels raised while continuing to breathe.

Suggested counterpose: Floor-Touch.

10. FLOOR-TOUCH (*Uttānāsana*)

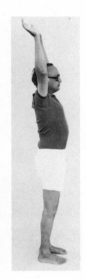

Exhale ↓

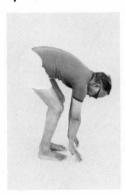

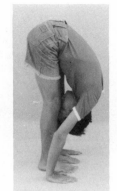

FINAL POSE

Suggested counterposes: Squat, Kneeling Bend, Knee Hold.

11. CANTILEVER (*Ardha Uttānāsana*)

Begin from   r-Touch.

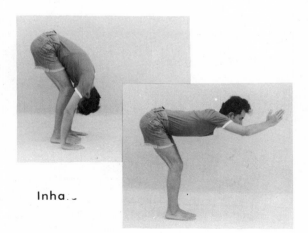

Inha._

Floor-Touch was the second asana of the Model Practice Sequence. See page 25 for instructions and page 35 for commentary.

After repeating several times, you may want to remain in the head-down, bent-knee position for several breaths.

In the final pose, the forehead touches the legs without their having to bend. Palms rest on the floor.

Inhaling,   ng the knees bent, come up part way wl   traightening the back. Lift the arms, pa   gether, and look up.

51

Exhaling, return the palms to the floor.

After several repetitions you may stay several breaths in Cantilever.

In the final position, the legs are straight, forming a right angle with the trunk.

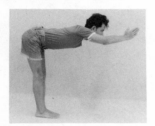

Suggested counterposes: Squat, Bridge, Knee Hold.

12. SQUAT (*Utkaṭāsana*)

Stand with feet together or slightly spread. Inhaling, lift the arms.

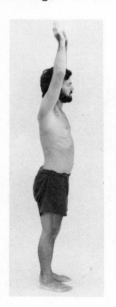

Exhale

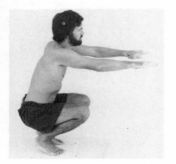

Exhaling, slowly sit down on the heels, lowering the arms part way.

Inhaling, rise up.

After several repetitions, you may pause for a few breaths in the squatting position.

In the classic pose, the heels do not leave the floor, and the arms remain extended overhead.

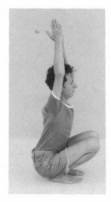

Suggested counterposes: Floor-Touch, Knee Hold, Supine Rest.

13. SPREAD-LEG FLOOR-TOUCH (*Prasārita-Pāda Uttānāsana*)

This is similar to Floor-Touch, but with the legs spread 2½ to 4 feet apart.

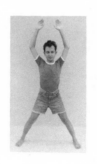
Exhale

Exhaling, slowly bend over and touch the floor. Bend the knees as necessary.

Inhaling, come up.

Repeat several times. Stay several breaths if you wish.

You will have attained the final pose when, with feet spread farther apart, you can bring the head to the floor and straighten the legs.

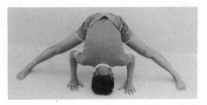

Suggested counterposes: Floor-Touch, Squat, Kneeling Bend, Knee Hold.

14. SIDE STRETCH (*Prasārita-Pāda Pārshwa Tānāsana*)

Stand with legs spread. Interlock the fingers, palms in or out as you prefer.

Inhaling, lift the arms overhead.

Exhaling, stretch the trunk sideways. Turn the head gently upward, i.e., if you are stretching toward the left side, turn the head toward the right arm.

Inhaling, return to Position 2.

Exhale as you lower the arms to Position 1.

Repeat this procedure to the other side. After several cycles you can pause for several breaths in Position 3. Be sure to do likewise on the other side.

Suggested counterposes: Spread-Leg Floor-Touch, Floor-Touch.

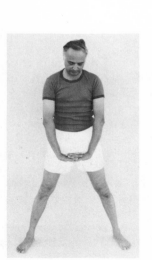

Inhale ➞

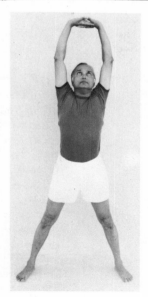

Exhale ➞

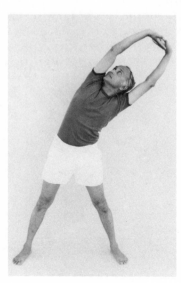

15. TRIANGLE TWIST (*Utthita Trikonāsana*)

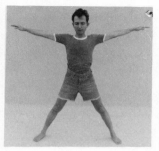

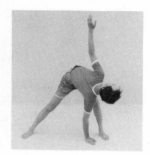

Triangle Twist was the third member of the Model Practice Sequence. See page 25 for instructions and pages 35-37 for commentary.

As you become comfortable in the pose you may wish to stay in it for more than the one breath suggested in Chapter 3. If so, stay the same number of breaths when you have twisted to the other side.

In the classic pose, both legs are straight and the hand is placed on the floor to the far side of the foot.

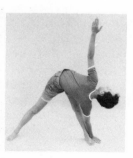

Suggested counterposes: Spread-Leg Floor-Touch, Floor-Touch, Kneeling Bend.

16. STRIDING STRETCH (*Pārshwa Uttānāsana*)

Stand with feet together and arms at sides. Step forward so that about a yard separates the feet (more or less, depending on your height). Turn the rear foot outward by about 45 degrees. Inhaling, raise the arms.

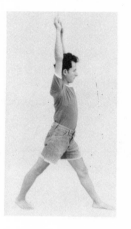

Exhale

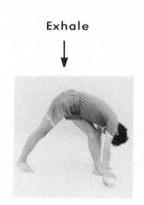

Exhaling, slowly bend over and touch the floor. The leg in front may bend.

Inhaling, come up.

Repeat several times. Stay down an additional few breaths if you are comfortable in the pose.

Come up as you inhale; lower arms as you exhale.

Bring the feet back together; then step forward with the other leg. Do the asana in the identical way on this side.

In the final pose, the front leg is straight, and the head is brought to touch it. Palms rest on the floor.

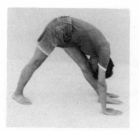

Suggested counterposes: Kneeling Bend, Floor-Touch, Squat.

17. FENCER (*Vīrabhadrāsana*)

Fencer starts like Striding Stretch, only the stride is deeper. Inhaling, raise the arms.

Bend down, exhaling and allowing the front knee to bend.

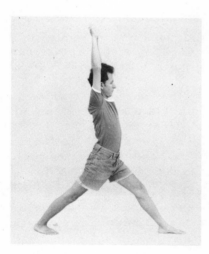

Then, inhaling, further bend the front leg, glide forward, lift the trunk, and raise the arms overhead. (For safety's sake, the arms should remain a little forward of the ears.)

Exhale

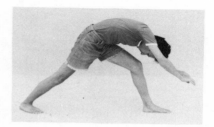

Inhale

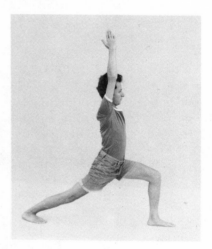

Exhaling, return to Position 2. Move several times between Positions 2 and 3. Then, if you wish, stay in Position 3 for several breaths. To switch sides, exhale to Position 2, inhale to Position 1, and exhale, lowering the arms. Bring the feet together, step forward with the other leg, and do asana in the identical way.

Suggested counterposes: Floor-Touch, Knee Hold.

18. UMBRELLA (*Vīrabhadrāsana variation*)

Umbrella begins from Fencer.

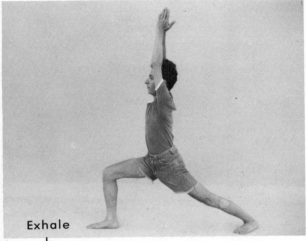

Exhale

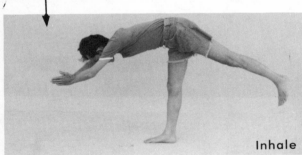

Inhale

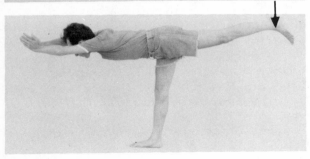

Exhaling, shift your weight onto the front leg, lift the rear foot, and straighten the supporting leg.

Inhaling, lift the rear leg, the chest and the arms.

Relax to Position 2 on exhalation. Repeat. After some practice you may attempt to stay in the final pose for several breaths.

To come out of the pose, reverse the movements and breathing; then follow the directions for coming out of Fencer. Step together, advance the other leg, and do the asana in the identical way.

Suggested counterposes: Squat, Knee Hold.

ASANAS ON "ALL-FOURS"

19. QUADRUPED [*Chakravākāsana*]

In the Model Practice Sequence, a three-step version of Quadruped served as counterpose to Triangle Twist. We give here a simpler version.

Kneel on the mat; the knees may be several inches apart. Place hands on the mat about two feet in front of the knees (more or less depending on your height), so that arms and thighs are perpendicular to the mat. Spread the hands so that the wrists are directly under the shoulders. Slightly bend the elbows.

Exhale and glide backward. Try to arch the back from hips to head. Lower the head and elbows part way toward the mat.

Inhale and glide forward, gradually straightening the arms. Let your back go hollow. Lift the chin.

Move several times between Positions 2 and 3. Either position may then be held for an additional few breaths.

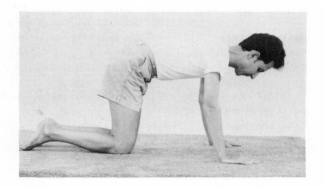

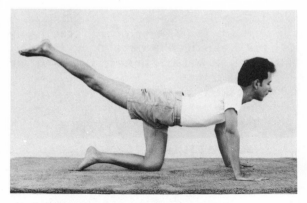

Suggested counterpose: Kneeling Bend.

20. PYRAMID (*Adho-Mukha Shwānāsana*)

Pyramid may be approached in several ways. In this variation, it starts from Quadruped, Position 3, but with the pads of the toes on the floor.

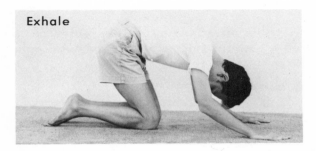

Exhale

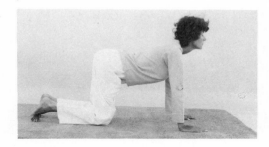

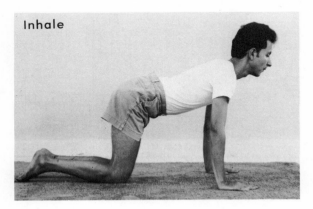

Inhale

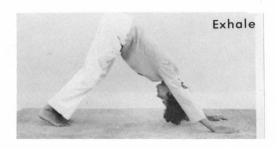

Exhale

In the classic Chakravakasana, one leg is extended and held high.

Exhaling, lift the knees and straighten the legs as much as you comfortably can. Lower the head. Keep the elbows relaxed.

Inhaling, lower the knees to the mat and resume Quadruped.

Repeat a few times to limber up. Then stay in Pyramid for several breaths.

Suggested counterpose: Quadruped.

SITTING ASANAS

The following nine asanas include some rudimentary sitting postures, as well as movements which help develop the flexibility and strength necessary to stay in them.

21. KNEELING BEND (*Vajrāsana*)

Version 1:

Kneel on the mat with arms at sides. Inhaling, raise the arms overhead.

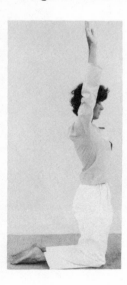

Exhale

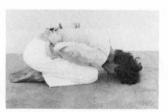

Exhaling, sit back toward the heels as you bend the trunk forward. Meanwhile, with elbows bent, sweep the arms down, out to the sides, and behind. The hands come to rest against the back.

Inhaling, lift the trunk, straighten up to the kneeling position, and sweep the arms outward, forward, and upward.

Move several times between the two positions. Then, if you like, you may remain crouched for several breaths.

Version 2:

In this variation you remain seated on the heels. Lock the fingers behind the back, palms out or in.

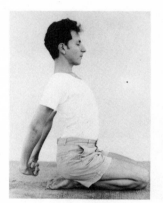

Exhale

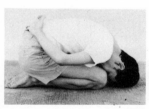

As you exhale, bend forward, and at the same time bend the elbows. Inhaling, sit up straight and stretch the arms behind you.

Repeat several times. Remain crouched for several breaths if desired.

Version 3:

Sit on the heels with arms at sides. Inhaling, raise the arms and press the palms together.

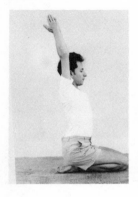

Exhale

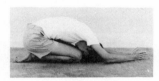

Exhaling, bend forward. Ideally your hands will not touch the mat until after your head does.

Inhaling, lift the arms first (if possible), then the head, and sit up.

Repeat the movement several times. Hold the pose several breaths.

Suggested counterposes: Table, Supine Rest.

22. TABLE (*Chatush-Pāda Pīṭha*)

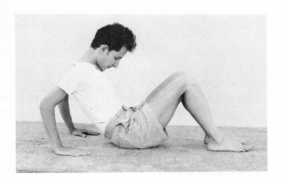

Inhale

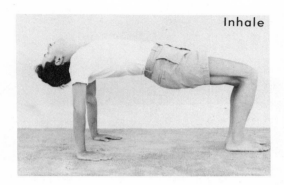

In the Model Practice Sequence, the Table pose functioned as a complement to Sitting Stretch. See page 35 for instructions and pages 41-42 for commentary. Like most asanas, in addition to being performed dynamically, Table may also be maintained for several breaths.

Suggested counterpose: Knee Hold.

23. SITTING STRETCH (*Pashchimatānāsana*)

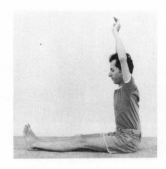

Exhale

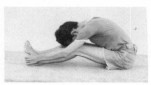

Sitting Stretch came toward the end of the Model Practice Sequence. See page 29 for instructions and page 41 for commentary. As explained there, allowing the legs to bend facilitates stretching the back. To stay in the pose, hold the legs wherever most convenient. For example, you may, as in the photograph, hold the sides of the feet.

The final position is reached when the legs no longer have to be bent in order for the head to rest on them.

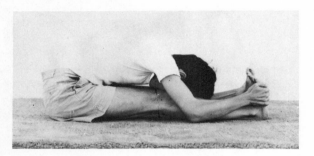

Suggested counterposes: Table, Knee Hold.

24. BOOK END [*Daṇḍāsana*]

The final position in Book End looks like the initial position in Sitting Stretch.

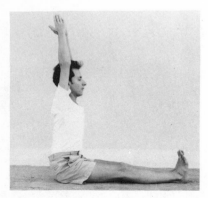

Since sitting erect with legs straight may be difficult for you, we offer two dynamic variations.

Version 1:

Sit with legs slightly bent and arms at sides.

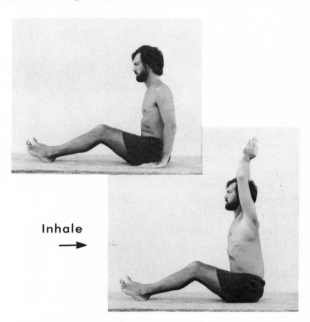

Inhale
→

Inhaling, raise the arms and try to straighten the back. Then, exhaling, lower the arms and relax.

Version 2:

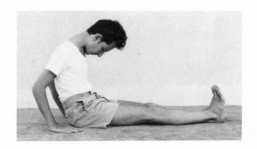

60

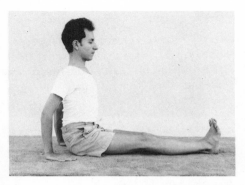

Straighten the back on each inhalation, as in Version 1, but this time with hands on the mat, just behind and to the sides of the hips.

You may stay for several breaths in either version, as in the final pose.

Suggested counterposes: Sitting Stretch, Knee Hold, Bridge.

25. ONE-LEG STRETCH (*Jānu shīrshāsana*)

One-Leg Stretch is useful as a preparation or substitute for Sitting Stretch. It helps loosen the hips, and allows you to work equally on each of the legs and on each side of the back.

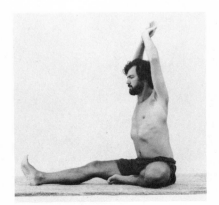

Exhale →

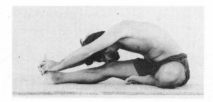

The technique is identical to Sitting Stretch, except that you sit with one foot against the other thigh. Repeat the asana for the same number of breaths with leg position reversed.

In the final position, the flexion is deeper and the extended leg is unbent.

Suggested counterposes: Table, Knee Hold.

26. SPREAD-LEG STRETCH (*Upaviṣhtha Konāsana*)

Sit with legs spread apart. Inhaling, lift the arms overhead.

Version 1:

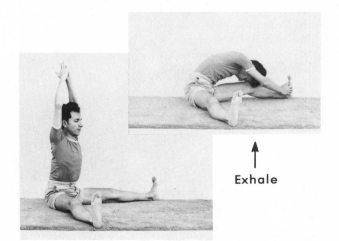

↑
Exhale

Exhaling, turn and bend the trunk toward one of the legs. Bend the leg if necessary.

Inhaling, come up.

Exhaling again, turn and bend to the other side.

Do several cycles. If you want to remain in the posture, hold the sides of the foot. Stay for the same number of breaths when holding the other foot.

Version 2:

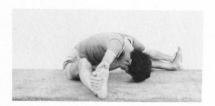

Exhale as you bend forward between the legs. Bend them if necessary.

Inhaling, come up.

Repeat as desired. To stay in the pose, hold the sides of the feet.

In the final position, the head touches the mat, the legs remain unbent, and the arms are extended with palms pressed.

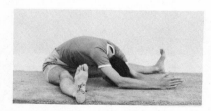

Suggested counterposes: Table, Knee Hold.

27. SITTING TWIST (*Ardha Matsyendrāsana*)

Kneel on the mat and sit on your heels. Place one hand—let us say the right one—behind the back. Cup your left hand over the outside of the right knee.

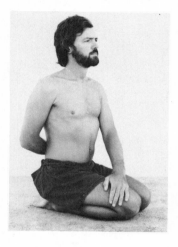

Exhale

↓

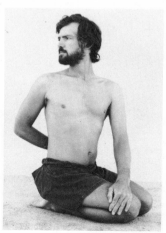

Exhaling, turn toward the right side. Begin the twisting at the level of the hips and finish by turning the right shoulder and the head.

Inhaling, return to Position 1.

Repeat several times. Then reverse the arms and twist to the other side for the same number of breaths.

You may be familiar with a different Sitting Twist; there are many variations. In most of the ways in which it is possible to sit, it is also possible to twist. However, the classic expressions of Ardha Matsyendrasana, including the one shown below, are impractical for most beginners.

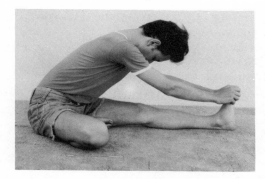

However, a modified version of Maha Mudra, which we call Volcano, is practicable even for beginners and is an excellent exercise for strengthening the back.

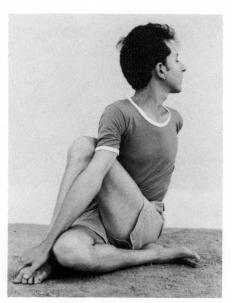

Suggested counterposes: Kneeling Bend, Sitting Stretch.

28. VOLCANO (Mahā Mudrā)

Mahā Mudrā is much praised in texts on Yoga. It is very arduous to maintain.

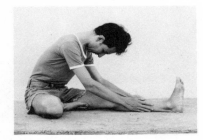

Inhale

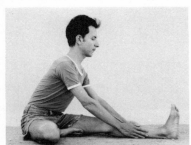

Sit as for One-Leg Stretch, with both hands holding the leg somewhere between the ankle and the knee—however you are most comfortable.

Inhaling, try to straighten the back. Keep the hands on the leg, the arms relaxed, and the elbows slightly bent.

Exhale in place.

Maintain the pose, trying to straighten the back a little more with each inhalation.

Reposition the legs and stay for the same number of breaths on the other side.

Suggested counterposes: Quadruped, Kneeling Bend, Knee Hold.

29. BOAT (*Nāvāsana*)

Sit as in Book End, Version 2, but with hands a little farther behind you. Inhale and straighten the back.

Version 1:

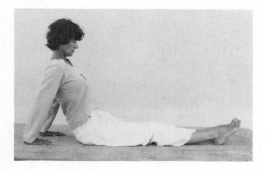

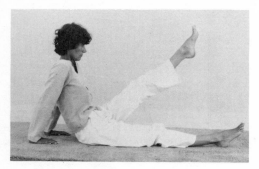

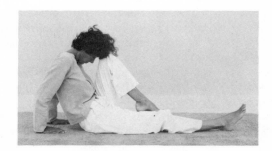

Exhaling, lift one leg, then bend it and bring the knee toward you.

Inhaling, stretch out the leg and lower it to the floor.

Then do likewise with the other leg. Do several cycles.

Version 2:

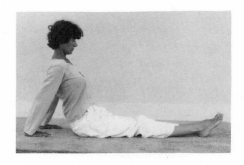

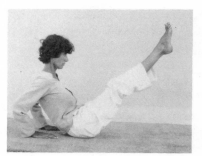

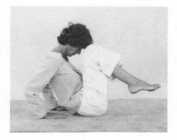

Exhale, lifting both legs, then bend them and bring the knees toward you.

Inhaling, stretch out the legs and lower them to the floor.

Repeat several times.

When, after some practice, you can lift the legs without needing to bend them, you can think of attempting the final pose shown below. It makes great demands on the legs, back, and abdomen.

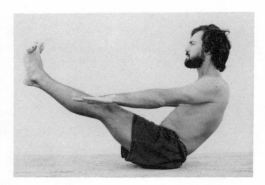

Suggested counterpose: Knee Hold.

PRONE ASANAS

The asanas in this group are excellent for strengthening the back. They are also good followups to Shoulderstand and its variations, which tend to compress the rib cage and the cervical vertebrae. If you suffer from chronic back pain, these prone asanas may not be advisable for the time being. Certainly, if you have trouble with these you should think twice before practicing more dramatic backbends.

30. COBRA (*Bhujaṅgāsana*)

Version 1:

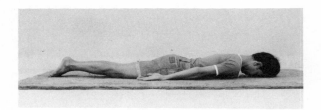

Inhale ↓

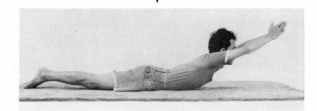

Cobra should be familiar from the Model Practice Sequence. See page 27 for instructions and page 40 for commentary. You can do the asana dynamically and you can also stay in the pose for several breaths. This is the classic form of Cobra, but you may want to try the following three variations, which have a slightly different effect and may be somewhat easier for you.

Version 2:

Place palms on the mat on either side of the chest, fingers pointing forward.

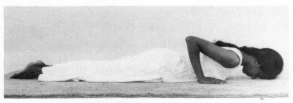

Inhale →

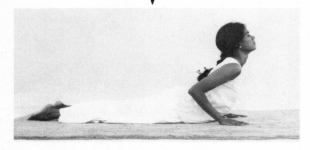

Inhaling, lift the chest off the mat. Don't put weight on the arms; the hands are for stability, not to push with.

Exhaling, lower the chest to the mat.

Repeat several times; then stay in the pose an additional few breaths.

Version 3:

Place the forearms on the mat, hands alongside the shoulders.

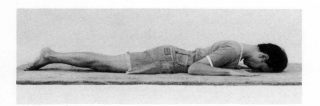

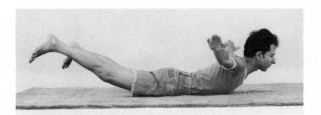

Inhale, lifting the chest off the mat. Lift and spread the arms at the same time.

Exhaling, retract the arms as you lower the chest.

Repeat several times, then stay.

Version 4:

Starting with arms at sides, bend the elbows and lock the fingers, palms out. Rest the hands on the back.

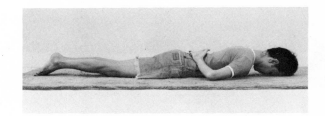

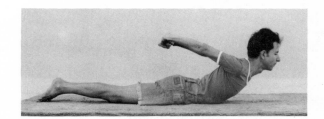

Inhaling, lift the chest and stretch the arms behind you. Fingers remain interlocked.

Exhaling, bring the hands to the back as you lower the chest.

Repeat and Stay.

Suggested counterposes: Knee Hold, Bridge, Kneeling Bend.

31. ARC (*Shalabhāsana*)

Shalabha is literally "grasshopper," but "Arc" seems more apt for the versions given here. Arc differs from Cobra in that the legs are lifted along with the chest. Since the fulcrum is shifted forward, Arc will not feel quite like Cobra. The three versions illustrated show how the pose may be practiced for varying effect.

Version 1:
Lie prone with arms at sides.

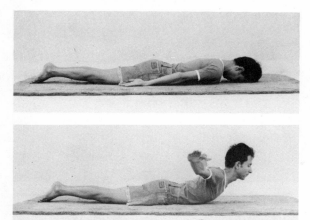

Inhaling, lift the legs, chest, and arms. Simultaneously spread the arms. You may also spread the legs.

Exhaling, simultaneously bring the legs together, lower them, bring the arms back to the sides, and lower the chest to the mat.

Repeat several times. Stay several breaths in the "flying" pose if you like.

Version 2:
First do Cobra, Version 1. Press the palms and maintain the pose while exhaling.

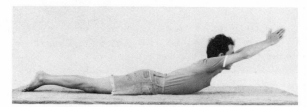

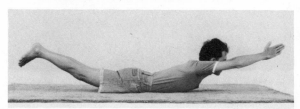

Inhaling, lift the legs.

Exhaling, lower the legs, keeping the chest off the floor.

Repeat several times.

To come out of the pose, lower chest as well as legs on an exhalation.

Version 3:
Lie prone with palms pressed.

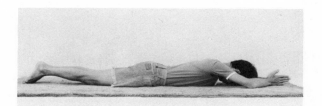

67

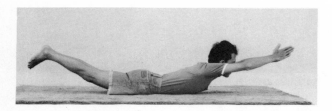

Inhaling, lift the legs, arms, and chest at the same time. Keep the palms pressed and straighten the arms.

Exhaling, lower the legs, arms, and chest to the mat.

Repeat several times. Then, if you like, you may stay in the pose for a few breaths more.

Suggested counterposes: Knee Hold, Bridge, Kneeling Bend.

32. SWIMMER (*Ardha Shalabhāsana*)

Swimmer is derived from Arc. It enables you to work on each side of the body separately. Lie prone with arms at sides. Inhaling, bring one arm forward and rest it on the mat.

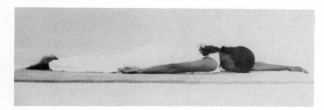

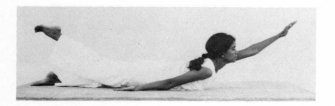

Inhaling, simultaneously lift the forward arm, the chest, and one leg. (The other arm remains at your side, the back of the hand against the mat.)

Exhaling, lower the arm, chest, and leg.

Repeat several times, lifting the legs alternately. Then do the movement the same number of times with arms reversed. If you want to stay in Swimmer, stay for the same number of breaths on each side.

Suggested counterposes: Knee Hold, Bridge, Kneeling Bend.

INVERTED ASANAS

33. SHOULDERSTAND (*Sarvāṅgāsana*)

Shoulderstand was included in the Model Practice Sequence (see page 28), and was discussed on pages 38-40.

Suggested counterposes: Supine Rest; then Cobra, Swimmer, or Arc.

34. HALF SHOULDERSTAND (*Viparīta Karaṇi*)

You may find this pose useful if you are too stiff to do Shoulderstand proper. Begin by lying on your mat with arms at sides.

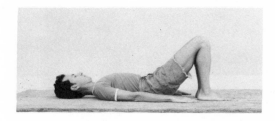

Exhaling, press the palms against the mat and lift the legs over the head. The legs should remain at roughly 45 degrees to the ground. The knees may be slightly bent.

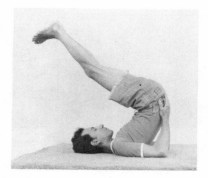

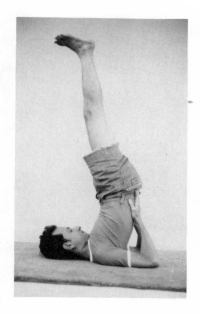

Stay in the pose with controlled breathing.

Whereas in Shoulderstand the body is supported primarily by the neck and shoulders, in Half Shoulderstand the weight is borne mostly by the upper back and arms. The legs should not be vertical, lest you strain the elbows.

If you still feel too much pressure on the elbows, lower the legs a little more. If you feel too much pressure on the head, slightly raise the legs. When your weight is properly distributed you should be able to lift the head momentarily off the mat.

Because of its different effect, Half Shoulderstand can be of value even if you can as easily do Shoulderstand. It is also a good substitute for Headstand.

Suggested counterposes: Bridge, Knee Hold, Supine Rest.

35. FOLDING SHOULDERSTAND (Ākunchanasana)

This variation was implied in the instructions for Shoulderstand on page 28. Easy leg movements will improve your stability in Shoulderstand.

First, go into Shoulderstand as before.

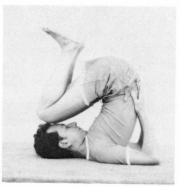

Exhaling, slowly bend and lower the legs. Inhaling, lift and stretch the legs.

Repeat as desired. You can also stay in the folded position for several breaths.

Suggested counterposes: Same as for Shoulderstand.

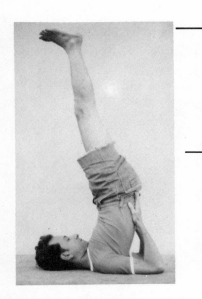 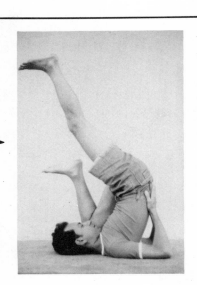 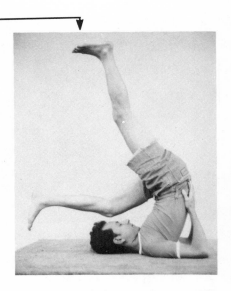

36. CYCLING SHOULDERSTAND (*Eka-Pāda Ākunchanāsana*)

This is a variant of the preceding. It will encourage an even development in both sides of the body and help keep your Shoulderstand from becoming lopsided.

Once again, start from Shoulderstand.

Exhaling, bend and lower one leg.

Inhaling, lift it back up.

Lower and lift the other leg in the same manner. Repeat the movement, alternating legs.

If you stay for several breaths with one leg flexed, be sure to do likewise with legs reversed.

Suggested counterposes: same as for Shoulderstand.

37. SPLIT-LEG SHOULDERSTAND (*Eka-Pāda Sarvāngāsana*)

Starting from Shoulderstand you again lower the legs in turn. This time the idea is to keep the legs straight, although you may bend them as much as necessary.

Exhaling, lower one leg as far as you can without losing control. The toes need not reach the floor.

Inhaling, lift the leg. Pressing the elbows firmly against the mat will help you maintain balance.

Exhaling, lower the other leg. Inhaling, lift it. Repeat several times in alternation.

When you can easily control the down and up movements of the leg you can try staying in the split-leg position for several breaths at a time each way.

Suggested counterposes: same as for Shoulderstand.

38. SPREAD-LEG SHOULDERSTAND (*Prasārita-Pāda Sarvānagāsana*)

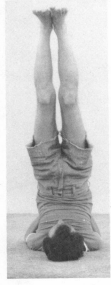

Front view
of
Shoulder Stand

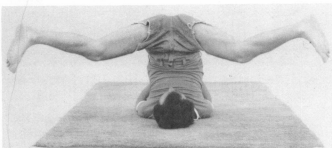

Exhaling, lower the legs slightly from Shoulderstand, spreading them outward at the same time.

Inhaling, bring the legs together as you lift them.

Repeat as desired. You may stay in the spread-leg position for several breaths.

Suggested counterposes: same as for Shoulderstand.

39. PLOUGH (*Halāsana*)

Plough begins from Shoulderstand. The first version is dynamic and preparatory. The second culminates in the static final pose.

Version 1:

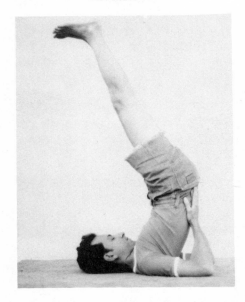

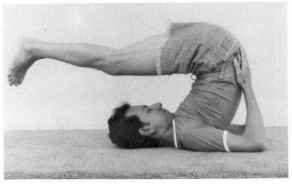

Exhaling, lower both legs, bending them as necessary.

Inhaling, lift the legs. This will be easier on the neck if you haven't lowered the toes all the way to the floor. Pressing the elbows also helps.

Lower and lift the legs several times. If you cannot easily *lift* both legs together, you shouldn't be *lowering* them—and are not yet ready for Plough. (For the time being, you can practice the Folding, Cycling, and Split-Leg variations of Shoulderstand described above.)

Version 2:

To reach the final position, begin from Shoulderstand.

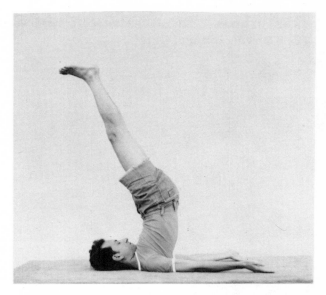

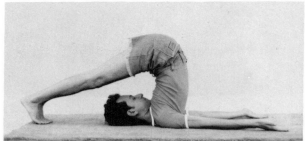

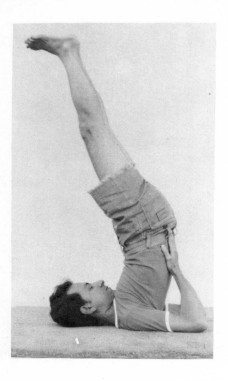

Exhaling, remove hand support, lower the forearms to the mat, and slowly lower the legs over the head. The toes may come to rest on the floor.

Stay several breaths.

To come out of the pose, bend the legs and roll out onto your back on an inhalation. (It isn't necessary to go back up into Shoulderstand first.)

Suggested counterposes: same as for Shoulderstand.

40. HEADSTAND (*Shīrṣhāsana*)

Headstand rightfully belongs in this collection, but it warrants a much fuller treatment than is possible here. Chapter 7 is devoted entirely to this very special asana.

6

YOGA AND THE BREATH

Discomfort...dejection...agitation...These are three sure signs of mental distraction. Yoga Sutra mentions a fourth: fitful breathing (I.31). One prescription for calming the mind is therefore "the conscious expulsion and retention of the breath" (I.34).

A present-day physician puts it this way: "A harmonious mind matches a rather slow and regular respiration; a troubled psyche speeds up the heart and breathing rhythms. All of us have experienced this occurrence whenever we pant or are short of breath because of some sudden emotion. The statement is reversible: a slow, harmonious, conscious breathing greatly promotes the mental faculties and the relaxation of the mind."[1]

Crucial as it is, we tend to ignore the breathing function until it stops performing normally and thrusts itself upon our consciousness. When we have a cold, or a bout of hay fever, or an asthmatic attack; when we get winded from physical exertion; when we are engulfed in smoke or noxious fumes; when we are stunned by emotional trauma—at these times we are painfully aware of our inability to breathe normally, and can appreciate the vital connection between breath and life. But this connection is always implicit in the view of Yoga, owing perhaps to the wider meaning of the Sanskrit word for "breath."

PRANA

Prāna, in a given context, might mean any of the following: "breath; wind; breath of air; vital air; vital spirit; vigor, energy, power; soul; intelligent principle; organ of sense."

The English word "breath," on the other hand, is descended from an Indo-European root meaning "make warm" (and is etymologically related to "breed," "brood," "brew," "broth," "bread," and "burn"). More akin to prana is the Latin *spiritus*, source of "spirit," "inspiration," "expiration," etc. Like prana, it conveys the idea of "life," "energy," and "invisible intelligence," thus demonstrating that the connection between these and "breath" is not really foreign to Western thinking.

Prana, therefore, is that which expresses our vitality, the quality of being alive. It is invisible and seemingly distinct from our physical body, yet no sooner do we lose the capacity to utilize it than that same precious body, not otherwise altered, becomes a worthless corpse, fit only for quick disposal.

Our breathing puts us into physico-chemical relationship with the world outside us. So do eating and drinking—but not as urgently, because we can do without food for days and water for hours. Like the food we eat, the air we breathe links us inseparably to the vegetable world. Oxygen makes possible the combustion of food fuels to release energy. Animals have evolved to take advantage of the oxygen liberated by the photosynthesis of growing plants, and depend on plants to reabsorb carbon dioxide.

The air we inhale does not belong to us any more than the currency notes we earn. Money in our possession is "ours" to spend, but once passed on to another, the same money becomes that person's property. Likewise, the air we breathe is ours to exploit, but once exhaled, the same molecules enter and reenter other organisms, animal and vegetable. We have life on loan. And even while we have it, it is not truly ours, since that life cannot be lived or conceived of except in intimate relation with all other life.

Vital as it is, breath is not the same as prana; it is an *index or manifestation of* prana As a physical discipline, Yoga aims at securing an optimum, interrelated functioning of the bodily systems. Prana, as represented by the breath, is essential to this functioning. But Yoga goes further in aspiring, by a profound increase in physical well-being, to bring about a more lucid, more harmonious functioning of the *mind.*

Mind and prana have a reciprocal, if elusive, relationship. Understood as energy and vitality, prana is dissipated when the mind is distracted. When the mind is calm and focused, prana is conserved. In aiming to restore mental clarity Yoga strives also to maximize prana. But Yoga recognizes that neither ob-jective can be tackled directly; we need an intermediary. It is through the medium of the breath that prana becomes accessible. The more confused we are, the more difficult it is for us to see through to the sources of our confusion; but even in relative confusion we can do something about our breathing.

The conscious effort to influence prana by means of breathing is known as *prāṇāyāma*. It is epitomized when we sit quietly and give full attention to the breath. But the attitude of pranayama pervades all of Yoga practice. It should be evident from the preceding chapters that asanas are immeasurably enriched by a simultaneous involvement with breathing.

Yoga is a practical science; where there is a theory there is also a technique. But before we consider the technique of breathing in Yoga, let us look at what happens physically when we breathe, and what we can do about it. The mechanics of respiration have been exhaustively described by physiologists; here we need only touch on the main points.

WHAT HAPPENS WHEN WE BREATHE

The principal organs of respiration are the paired lungs. They are the chambers in which deoxygenated blood from the heart comes into direct contact with oxygen-rich, freshly inhaled air. Oxygen is absorbed by the red blood cells and transported back to the heart, whence it is pumped through the arterial system to all the cells of the body. Meanwhile, carbon-dioxide laden blood returns via the veins to the heart to be pumped to the lungs. Excess CO_2 diffuses into the lungs and passes out of the body with the exhaled air.

The lungs have been likened to a pair of sponges or bellows. Their expansion and contraction is the direct result of pressure differentials between the thoracic, or chest, cavity—to whose inner wall they are attached by the intrapleural membrane—and the atmosphere outside the body. When the volume of the chest cavity is increased, internal pressure becomes negative and air is drawn into the lungs. Elastic recoil then initiates compression of the chest cavity, resulting in a positive internal pressure and expulsion of air through the windpipe.

Like all bodily movements, expansion and compression of the thorax result from muscular activity. The principal muscle of respiration is the diaphragm, which forms a convex partition between thorax and abdomen. Above the diaphragm are the heart and lungs; below it are the organs of digestion and other viscera. When stimulated, the diaphragm contracts downward, allowing the lower part of the lungs to inflate, and thereby accounting for at least two-thirds of their total expansion volume. At the end of inhalation the diaphragm relaxes and resumes its dome shape, squeezing air out of the lungs. (See the diagram on page 82.)

Besides the diaphragm, there are other breathing muscles, notably the intercostals. One set elevates and spreads the ribs, facilitating upper-lung expansion. The other set pulls the ribs downward and inward, compressing the lungs. However, during ordinary shallow breathing there is little need for contraction of the rib-cage muscles. Partial, involuntary contraction of the diaphragm creates a vacuum in the lungs sufficient to draw in air for the body's needs. Ventilatory rhythms are governed by a subtle complex of physical, chemical, emotional, and conditioned reflexes.

CONTROL OF BREATH

Like an airplane pilot switching off "automatic pilot" in favor of personal direction, we are free to assume conscious control of the breathing process. If the higher brain had to regulate breathing at all times, it would be unable to devote enough attention to more complicated tasks of information analysis and response. So, as long as body processes are functioning smoothly, it relies on automatic breath control—which is every bit as sophisticated as automatic flight control.

Yet, for all its advantages, automatic pilot is necessarily mechanical. Just as the pilot resumes active control when he is about to deviate from his course or altitude, or when weather conditions change, we may take over conscious breath control whenever it seems advantageous to do so.

Textbooks tell us that humans normally breathe at a rate of 12 to 20 cycles per minute. Inhalation and exhalation together, therefore, take approximately four seconds. Naturally, this rate would be sped up considerably by intense physical exertion, since increased muscular activity (including that of the heart) requres more O_2 for combustion and produces more CO_2 for elimination. Here is a case where the rate of breathing is best left to the body's automatic regulating devices. Any effort at curtailing that rate could be disastrous.

But suppose we are not engaged in strenuous exercise and are breathing peacefully. Isn't it still desirable to let the body maintain its own comfortable breathing rate? Would anything be gained, say, by deliberately *speeding up* that rate? Conceivably, if we felt very sluggish and drowsy, or had just emerged from a stuffy environment into fresh air, a few seconds of faster breathing might be invigorating. Any more than that, however, and we would begin to feel dizzy.

Now what of the other possibility? What if we purposely try to *slow down* the rate of breath? Before pursuing this line of inquiry we should note that slower breathing tends to encourage *deeper* breathing. If we take more time to fill and empty the lungs we will move a greater volume of air. So a parallel question arises: What are the advantages, if any, to breathing more deeply—more deeply than the body says we need to be breathing?

Surely all of us have noticed how a few deep breaths can calm the mind. But how is it that we catch ourselves breathing too quickly or too shallowly in the first place? If a little slow breathing makes us feel so much better, why should it require conscious intervention? In order to account for this paradox we need to look more closely at the mechanism of involuntary breath regulation.

BREATHING AND THE FIGHT/FLIGHT RESPONSE

Of the two branches of the autonomic nervous system, it is the *sympathetic* which mobilizes the body in response to alarm. The pattern of signals it triggers has become popularly known as the "fight or flight" response. Whether we choose to fight or to flee is up to the higher brain, where all relevant sensory and recollected information is rapidly processed. What the sympathetic system does is to gear us physiologically for either course of action.

When the fight/flight response is elicited by the imminence of peril, all sorts of preparedness adjustments are swiftly made. One of these is a rapid increase in cardiac and respiratory rates. Whether we fight or flee,

we are going to make a concerted demand on our muscles. They will need all the oxygen they can get, and their contractions will produce carbon dioxide. Rapid ventilation, deeper than normal, will accelerate gaseous exchange in the lungs. More vigorous circulation will insure that the blood can accommodate the gas and adequately service the muscles.

Kurt Vonnegut has given us an engaging clinical description of this process:

My mind sent a message to my hypothalamus, told it to release the hormone CRF into the short vessels connecting my hypothalamus and my pituitary gland.

The CRF inspired my pituitary gland to dump the hormone ACTH into my bloodstream. My pituitary had been making and storing ACTH for just such an occasion....

And some of the ACTH in my bloodstream reached the outer shell of my adrenal gland, which had been making and storing glucocorticoids for emergencies. My adrenal gland added the glucocorticoids to my bloodstream. They went all over my body, changing glycogen into glucose. Glucose was muscle food. It would help me fight like a wildcat or run like a deer....

My adrenal gland gave me a shot of adrenaline, too. I turned purple as my blood pressure skyrocketed. The adrenaline made my heart go like a burglar alarm. It also stood my hair on end. It also caused coagulants to pour into my bloodstream, so, in case I was wounded, my vital juices wouldn't drain away.[2]

The fight/flight response makes it possible for us to react quickly to emergencies. The problem arises because the autonomic system—not being subject to our higher, more discriminating human intelligence—can't tell the difference between conditions of *danger* and conditions of *stress*. Let there be a threat to our emotional equilibrium and in no time the sympathetic system has our engines racing. Nerve impulses course through the body. Air is sucked in and expelled. Like an engine, warmed up and idling, we are humming and shaking and ready to go.

But if we go nowhere—if, instead of shifting into gear, we stand still, revving up over and over again—something is bound to go wrong in the engine. When during stressful periods we can neither fight nor flee, we are liable to all sorts of symptoms—migraines, ulcers, insomnia, hypertension. Stress is so common nowadays that it has come to seem the norm. What is worse, the effects of stress become causes of further stress.

When the urgency for fight or flight has passed, the complementary arm of the autonomic system, the *para*sympathetic, takes over. It acts to restore *homeostasis*.

This means a stable, ideal level of body temperature, water content, blood sugar, and scores of other factors....Homeostasis determines how efficiently your body and especially your brain work. 'The mind,' said Sir Charles Sherrington, a great neurologist, 'is like a sheet of water reflecting the world, and the faithfulness of the image depends on how calm the surface lies.' Disturbances of the internal environment ruffle the image; for example, a small increase or decrease of blood sugar, as in diabetes or insulin shock, distorts our lucid mental pictures or even wipes them out. The parasympathetics work to prevent such

disturbances or to smooth out ripples after disturbances. When you are resting, under parasympathetic dominance, your heart beats placidly; your digestive system is active; your breathing is quiet; your pupils are narrowed (unless you are in the dark); and all the rest of it.[3]

The parasympathetic system is thus responsible for what has been dubbed "rest and recuperation,"[4] or "the Relaxation Response."[5] Working through different nerve channels, the parasympathetic reverses the effects of the sympathetic but, like the latter, it is a package of responses and is nominally removed from conscious control.

One of the chief results of parasympathetic excitation is the slowing down of cardio respiratory rates. Heart rate is not normally subject to direct control, but breathing certainly is. Might it not be possible, *by deliberately slowing down our breathing*, to induce the whole cascade of calming effects which constitute the parasympathetic package? In other words, if we make a point of breathing more slowly, more completely, more rhythmically, can we expect to experience also the accompanying *involuntary* results of parasympathetic excitation—notably a lowered heart rate and overall relaxation? Much experimental work still needs to be done before the claims of Yoga practitioners can be confirmed, but the evidence is persuasive. Relaxation is in the mind and the muscles, but slower, deeper breathing may well function as a catalyst in bringing it about.

DISTINCTIVENESS OF YOGA BREATHING

Before proceeding with our investigation of breathing, we should be clear on the distinction between *rate* of ventilation and *degree* of ventilation. Rate of ventilation is a measure of the number of breath cycles per unit of time. Degree of ventilation refers to the volume of the amount of expansion in the lungs. When we use adjectives like "slow" and "rapid," we are talking about rate; while degree of ventilation is expressed by words like "shallow" and "deep." The intersection of these variables in the types of breathing we have been discussing is shown in this table:

Type of Breathing	Rate of Ventilation	Degree of Ventilation
Normal	Slow	Shallow
Excited	Rapid	Deep
Yoga	Slower	Deeper

Terms like "slow" or "deep" are only relative. Normal breathing, legitimately described as "slow" in comparison to excited breathing, is not at all slow compared to Yoga. Similarly, excited breathing, though deeper than quiet breathing, is hardly as deep as Yoga breathing. A graphic representation of the above table might look like this:

VALUE OF YOGA BREATHING

Slow, deep breathing does more than just facilitate relaxation; it is tonic to the entire cardio-respiratory system. While easing stress and tension, it simultaneously exercises the heart and lungs in the safest, most effective manner, and progressively augments the body's resistance to potentially stressful situations.

Cardio-respiratory fitness depends in part on the efficiency of ventilation. Healthy, elastic lungs can expand more; lungs which expand more can take in more air with each breath; lungs which take in more air with each breath need take fewer breaths—and, in the process, become healthier and more elastic.

Ventilation, of course, is not a closed system; it operates in tandem with circulation. The chief organ of the circulatory system—the heart—has an absolutely vital function. It sends the blood through a branching network of tubes, and must maintain a pressure high enough for all the cells of the body to be

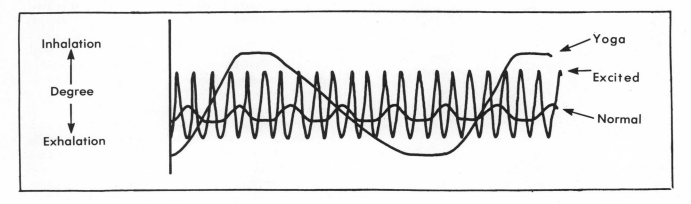

adequately supplied with nutrients and relieved of wastes. The heart pumps reliably through every minute of our lives; when it can no longer do so life ceases. Wear and tear on the heart is reduced by better breathing. Efficient lungs bring more oxygen into contact with the blood sent to them by the heart, resulting in a richer arterial blood supply. When the oxygen-carrying capacity of the blood is more fully utilized, the heart needn't work as hard to get oxygen to the tissues.

Yoga breathing also lessens the work of the heart by maximizing pressure differentials.

> The circulation of blood in the lungs is maintained by the heart beats, and is made easier by the movements of inhalation and exhalation. In fact, during inhalation, a negative pressure is produced, promoting the flow of blood from the neck and from the abdomen to the heart, and hence to the lungs. The endopulmonary pressure is reversed and becomes positive during exhalation, thus promoting the expulsion of the blood oxygenated in the lungs. One can easily understand this mechanism by comparing the thorax to a hand holding a sponge immersed in the water: when the hand opens, the sponge expands; when it closes the sponge is squeezed.[6]

The more the sponge is squeezed, the more water is expelled.

So it is with the lungs. The deeper the inhalation, the greater the negative-pressure effect, drawing blood back to the heart through the veins and then on to the lungs. The deeper the exhalation, the greater the positive-pressure effect, expelling oxygenated blood back to the heart for distribution to the cells through the arterial system. When the blood is already under significant pressure because of lung activity, the heart does not have to labor very hard to boost that pressure to the required levels. Indeed, the powerful rhythmic suction of the lungs provides a marvelous exercise to the heart muscle, improving its tone while at the same time relieving it of strain.

A healthier heart shows up not merely in freedom from heart-related disease, but in the reduction of excessive blood pressure and heart rate, and in the steadying and strengthening of the cardiac contractions. A complete heart-beat cycle comprises a contraction, lasting less than half a second; followed by a relaxation, during which blood fills the chambers of the heart and flows through its vessels. The healthy heart which can afford to beat less frequently enjoys longer intervals of rest.

The practice of Yoga breathing, even for short periods, provides a physical and a psychological pickup. Little by little it supplants lazy breathing habits with healthier ones. Left to itself, the body often follows the path of least resistance, preferring bad habits to good innovations. A rate of 12-20 breaths per minute may indeed be "normal," but this may be, not so much the optimal range for persons of exuberant health, as the average for persons of indifferent health. The idea behind the exercise of good breathing habits during Yoga practice is for these habits to carry over into ordinary unconscious breathing as well.

TECHNIQUE OF YOGA BREATHING

Having discussed the "what-is" of Yoga breathing, let us turn our attention to the "how-to." As might be expected, there is more consensus as to theory than method. The method recommended here is not the only one in use; possibly you have been taught to breathe in a different manner. All that is asked is that you examine it critically and experiment with it. By all means reject any part of it that doesn't feel right to you.

All breathing, as we have seen, depends on the action of specific muscles. If you want to alter your manner of breathing you must develop greater control over those muscles. They can be exercised like any other muscles. Like other muscles, they are not called into play directly but by your concentrating on the work you want performed. While it may be of academic interest to know which muscle groups are responsible for which movements, it is no use trying to invoke a particular muscle. Your nervous system makes that decision for you after you decide what you want done.

HOW TO INHALE

When it comes to breathing, what do you want done? First of all, you want to be sure the diaphragm is contracting fully, in order to permit maximum expansion of the lower lobes of the lungs. As it happens, you cannot will the contraction of the diaphragm. But really you don't need to. All you need do is slow down the rate of inhalation to allow the diaphragm time to contract fully. Deliberately pushing the abdomen forward and outward may reinforce the feeling of expansion, but it is of questionable utility in promoting greater filling of the lungs. In any case, however much you push out your abdomen, you should certainly not pull it in! Doing so would definitely inhibit the diaphragm.

Possibly you have been told to "pull the air all the way down" to the navel or even the groin. While conceptualizing thus may have the desired effect, it is physiologically inaccurate. The destination of the air is the lungs, which descend only as far as the lowest ribs. The region below the diaphragm is filled with digestive and eliminative—not respiratory—organs.

As was mentioned earlier, the lifting and spreading of the ribs account for a much smaller increase in lung volume than does contraction of the diaphragm, but these are indispensable to Yoga breathing. In many persons rib-cage expansion tends to be negligible unless consciously initiated. One reason is that the powerful diaphragm muscle, on contracting, pulls against the lower ribs, to which it is attached, effectively preventing them from spreading further. Another impediment to the lifting of the ribs is the force of gravity (at least in upright postures). You can counteract gravity, but not without some effort. This effort must progress from the top downward, since the external intercostal muscles work by pulling each rib toward the previously elevated and fixed rib above it.

Though the diaphragm and chest components are equally important, which one you concentrate on depends upon your prior habits. If you are a belly breather you should devote more attention to first lifting and spreading the ribs. If you are a chest breather try to relax more and let the diaphragm descend fully. As to sequence, the general rule is that conscious muscular activity in inhaling *begins in the chest* and *ends in the abdomen*.

Attention to the chest during inhalation encourages maintenance of an erect spinal column and strengthens the postural muscles of the back. By contrast, initiating the breath at the level of the abdomen allows the upper back to remain slumped for a longer interval and contributes to neck strain.

HOW TO EXHALE

As you exhale the diaphragm relaxes and pushes up the chest floor, while the ribs draw inward and downward. Thus the lungs are compressed from all sides. The order of events is simply the reverse of inhalation.

Whereas expanding the rib cage required conscious effort, collapsing it requires none. Rather, you should try to maintain the expansion as long as possible into the exhalation, in order to permit the back to remain erect a little longer. The diaphragm will relax by itself, but contracting the abdominal muscles helps to control and deepen the exhalation. Meanwhile, the rib cage will collapse without your having to help it along.

Complete exhalation, therefore, requires attention primarily to the abdomen. Allowing the belly to puff out or protrude is not only technically wrong but unhealthy. It may accompany a tendency to suck the belly in on inhalation, which would interfere with the descent of the diaphragm and the filling of the lower lungs. If you discover that you have this tendency you should strive to counteract it. In your case, there is probably too much happening in the upper chest by way of compensation, so you need not try to lift the ribs still further. Concentrate exclusively on the abdomen until you have developed proper coordination.

If the foregoing analysis seems too involved, you need only remember that the volume of air you take in can be no more than the space you provide for it. The more you enlarge the thorax—in every dimension—the more the lungs are stretched, and the more air is drawn in to fill the vacuum. The more you compress the thorax, the more the lungs are squeezed and the more complete is the expulsion of air.

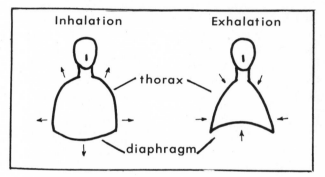

PLACEMENT OF THE BREATH

Try to use your nose for breathing. True, air can as well enter through the mouth, but only in the nose is it properly filtered. Chronic mouth breathing dries out the throat and weakens your resistance to respiratory infection. Furthermore, it is not as easy to control the breath through the mouth, and controlled breathing is what we are after in Yoga. At times you have no choice but to breathe through the mouth—as when swimming, or when your nose is congested. But as a rule, nose breathing is preferable, and the practice of Yoga will encourage it.

As your breath becomes more refined, you will begin to sense it in the region of the throat. Of course, the air will still be passing through the nostrils, but too gently to be producing a noise there. Instead you will become aware of a faint frictional sound within the pharynx. This "throat sound," as we shall be referring to it, will come about on its own, as your breathing in asanas becomes slower and more uniform.

Once you get the knack of throat-sound breathing you should avoid exaggerating it. The sound need only be loud enough to be audible to you, so that you can use your hearing faculty to help monitor the steadiness of the breath. The finer your breathing, the subtler will be the sound. If you can be conscious of the breath in the throat without its causing any sound at all, so much the better.

BREATHING IN ASANAS: A REVIEW

In Chapter 8 we shall see how Yoga breathing finds its fruition in the practice of pranayama. But here let us recapitulate some of the arguments for doing Yoga breathing even in asanas—in static as well as dynamic variations. If pranayama is the fruit of Yoga breathing, asana is the flower from which it emerges.

Without claiming to be exhaustive, we can affirm that breathing in asanas:

1. Exercises deeper layers of muscle
2. Distributes the exercise more evenly between muscles and joints.
3. Guards against fatigue, overexertion
3. Guards against fatigue, overexertion, and strain.
4. More completely ventialtes the lungs.
5. Increases the active participation of chest and upper back.
6. More deeply massages the abdominal viscera.
7. Lessens the load on the heart.
8. More efficiently circulates the blood throughout the body
throughout the body.
9. Yields deeper relaxation.
10. Keeps postures from becoming tedious or mechanical.
11. Encourages greater presence of mind in the affairs of the body.
12. Leads naturally to breathing in pranayama.

7

HEADSTAND: HOW AND WHY

If you mention that you practice Yoga someone is sure to ask you whether you stand on your head. What is so special about Headstand (*Shīrshāsana*)? Why is it associated with Yoga? In this chapter we shall look impartially at this curious and controversial asana. But first let us be clear as to what we mean by Headstand. What is it and how is it done?

TECHNIQUE

The following is a fail-safe procedure for attaining the pose. There are ten steps. It may take you days or years to reach the advanced stages. If you are intent on learning Headstand you should not rely solely on this or any other book but should seek instruction from an expert. All we claim is that the ten-step method here recommended will take you gradually and safely toward the final pose. Each step leads to the next. If, for example, Step 5 is too difficult for you, it is unlikely you could do Step 8 correctly.

It is possible to learn Headstand without using a wall for support, even in the initial stages. But for most people a wall is a great help, so in our method it is not until Step 10 that wall support is dispensed with. Only when you can do all the preceding steps should you attempt Headstand away from a wall.

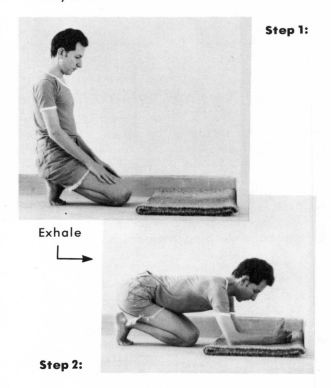

Step 1:

Exhale

Step 2:

84

Place a mat—thick but not spongy—against an empty wall. Sit on your heels facing the wall, with knees and toes on the floor.

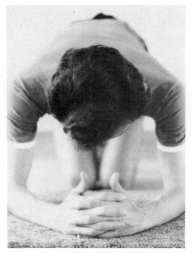

Exhaling, bend forward slowly. Interlock the fingers and place the hands on the mat, 3 or 4 inches from the base of the wall. (Only the edge of the hand rests on the mat—not the knuckles.) Position the forearms on the mat so that the elbows are spread as far apart as your shoulders. Then, for added stability, you may spread the elbows a little farther apart.

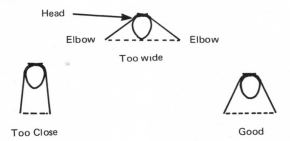

Extend the thumbs upward. Place the head on the mat, cradled by the hands, thumbs pressing firmly against the back of the skull.

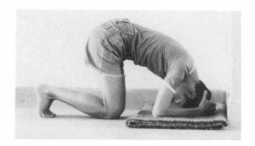

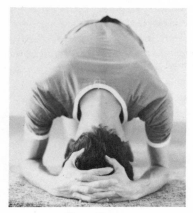

Front View

You will learn by trial and error what spot on the skull should rest on the mat. It can be determined by imagining two plumb lines bisecting your body from front and side, while you are standing on your feet in a balanced carriage. Since you cannot see the top of your head, you might ask your teacher to look at you and mark approximately where the lines meet on the skull.

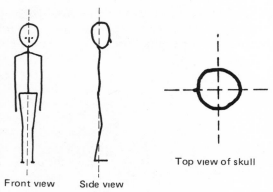

Front view   Side view

Top view of skull

Keep in mind, when positioning the head on the mat, that the head will roll slightly as you go up into Headstand. Thus you should place the head, in Step 2, so that the point of contact is somewhat nearer the forehead than you want it to be when you are fully inverted.

Check also that your legs are symmetrically aligned. Spread the knees apart so that you can see the toes. Your line of vision should be perpendicular to an imagined line connecting the elbows.

(Viewed from above)

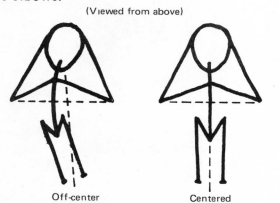

Off-center   Centered

Pause for a few breaths in Step 2. If you feel dizzy or are not sure that you are correctly positioned, do not proceed further.

Step 3:

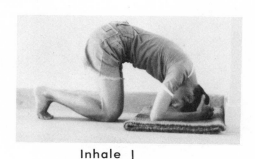

Inhale

Inhaling, lift your knees off the floor.

Step 4:

Exhale

86

Exhaling, slowly tiptoe forward. Your weight will shift gradually in the direction of the wall; compensate by firmly anchoring the elbows. If you find difficulty in doing so, or if your arms begin to tremble, go no further. Even with toes still on the ground your trunk is already substantially inverted. If you are uncomfortable physically or mentally, there is no point in going beyond Step 4.

Step 5:

After exhaling

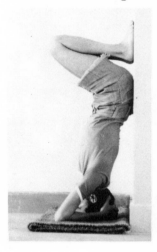

Between breaths—i.e., having exhaled but before inhaling—press the elbows, push off with the toes, and bring the feet to the wall. The legs are still bent, but in all essential respects you are in Headstand. Stay in this position as long as you are steady and relaxed.

Be sure your forearms are in contact with the mat from elbows to hands, without a gap at the wrists. The interlocked fingers should not be tense. Are you still centered? Has your head tilted? Do you feel any pain at the neck? Is breathing a problem? If all is not in order you should come back down.

Now pay more attention to your breathing and see if you can deepen it. Don't be in a hurry to stretch the legs upward. Only when you can stay a couple of minutes in Step 5 with deep, relaxed breathing should you attempt to go further. It may be days or weeks before this is the case, but there's no rush: you are already getting all the important benefits of Headstand. The remaining steps are concerned mostly with perfecting the form.

Step 6:

Inhale

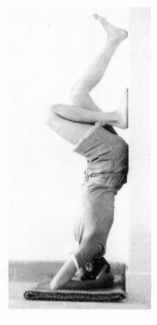

Inhaling, slowly extend one leg—let us say the left—sliding the heel up the wall. Don't straighten the left leg completely, but keep the knee slightly bent. You may stay a few breaths.

Exhaling, slowly flex and retract the left leg. Again, you may stay a few breaths.

On a subsequent inhalation, extend the right leg in the same way. On an exhalation, retract it.

Stretching one leg at a time keeps your center of gravity from shifting too suddenly. Practicing this step for a while insures that both sides of the body are working equally, and will pay off when you get to Steps 7 and 8. If you prematurely extend both legs, they may be markedly askew and may disturb the alignment of the spinal column.

When you get used to having one leg extended against the wall you may go a step further.

Step 7:

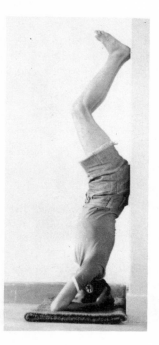

Inhaling, slowly stretch the other leg—in our example the right—sliding its heel up the wall so that it joins the left leg. You may stay a few breaths.

Step 8:

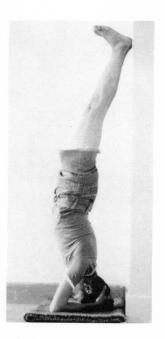

Inhaling, extend the legs, sliding the heels up the wall; press the elbows, and take the buttocks away from the wall.

Practicing against a wall allows you to test whether your body is straight. Inhaling, slide the heels apart along the wall until you feel that your left and right sides are balanced. Then, exhaling, inch the heels together, being careful to move them at an even rate.

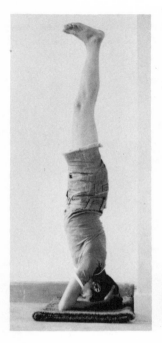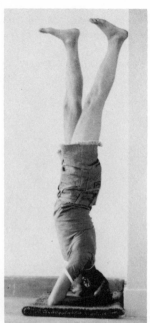

You may feel more secure in the pose if you keep the legs slightly spread.

Having advanced as far as Step 8 you should devote increasing attention to your breathing. Headstand is an excellent pose in which to work on the breath. As long as your breathing is deep and controlled it is safe to remain inverted—assuming of course that you feel no strain anywhere in the body. When you can easily stay for 16 breaths or four minutes—whichever is longer—you may begin practicing without wall support.

Step 9:

Exhaling, carefully remove the left heel from the wall. Stay a few breaths.

Inhaling, return the heel to the wall.

Do likewise with the right leg, while keeping the left heel against the wall.

When you are comfortable with one leg off the wall you may try with both.

Step 10:

Lift the left heel from the wall on exhalation, as in Step 9. Take one or two breaths.

On a subsequent exhalation, lift the right heel as well. Be sure your lateral alignment is not disturbed. Press the elbows to insure proper weight distribution. This is the final pose. Stay for a number of breaths.

After some practice you may be able to go directly to the final pose without having to rely on the wall. As in Step 8, the focus of attention is on the breath. Very likely you will discover it deepening. If, instead, it begins to speed up, or if you are uncomfortable or have doubts about your alignment, you should come down. After a few minutes, Headstand begins to have negative effects, even for the experienced practitioner. You mustn't assume that the longer you stay in it the better it is for you.

Bring the heels back to the wall one by one, on successive inhalations.

Make sure you have enough energy and control left to come out of the pose gracefully, by stages. If you crash to the floor you have obviously stayed too long. You should be able to move slowly through the ten steps in reverse sequence (with reverse breathing). However, by the time you are proficient enough to have gotten this far you can use this abbreviated sequence to descend:

Exhaling, bend both legs, sliding the heels down toward the buttocks.

Step 11:

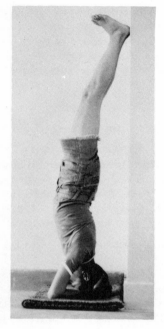

Step 13:

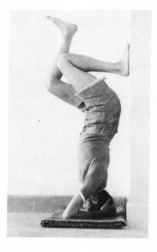

A

Inhaling, bring both heels back to the wall.

Step 12:

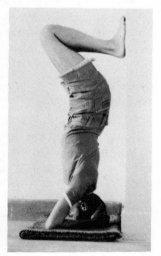

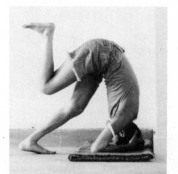

B

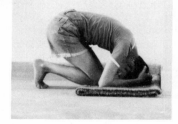

C

On the next exhalation, keeping both legs bent, lower one foot toward the floor. The second foot will follow of its own. This is the safest way down, though you can also bring both feet to the floor simultaneously.

Step 14:

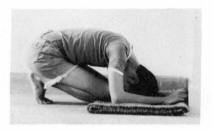

Once you are back on terra firma don't be in a hurry to get up. Release the hand grip and remain crouched a few breaths longer.

Then lie down on your back and rest. Your bones and muscles have been under an unaccustomed stress. The longer you were upside-down, the longer they will need to relax.

After resting for at least a minute you must do a counterpose for the neck. The counterpose par excellence is Shoulderstand.

ADVANTAGES

Headstand is obviously not to be attempted casually; it requires considerable attention. But why bother at all? What benefits does Headstand provide that are not obtainable by less extreme means?

In this and the next section I have borrowed and quoted liberally from a recent monograph by Dr. F. J. Chandra on "Medical and Physiological Aspects of Headstand."[1] Some of the findings are still provisional; although the value of Headstand has been recognized empirically for centuries, it has not yet received much scientific scrutiny.

The following advantages are surely not the only ones, but they have been particularly well-attested:

1. Blood drains from the legs.

With the effect of gravity reversed, a considerable volume of blood flows out of the legs. Blood pressure in the legs falls drastically, and swelling in the veins is reduced. The legs may not feel as heavy or tired after your practice.

2. Blood flow to the brain is improved.

With the body upended and blood draining from the legs toward the neck:

One might expect that this increased blood pressure would cause an influx of blood to the brain (which could cause problems). In fact this is not so, there is an auto-regulating mechanism in the brain to restrict the cerebral blood flow....

We think that the excess blood from the legs is diverted to muscles that are active, including those of the back, abdomen and arms, and the brain blood flow remains much the same. However one finds many claims that the head-down position has mental as well as physical effects. A majority of those who have been practicing headstand long enough to be accustomed to the position feel marked benefit from it. They report that after the posture they feel more clear mentally, have an improved memory, and have other beneficial effects. What might be the cause?...

What we think is that in the head-down position, where blood pressure in the neck is increased, but only temporarily, by about 20%, there is not an increased blood flow through the whole brain, but a general opening up of those blood vessels which were comparatively closed. Thus one net result after the headstand is probably a base-line opening of blood vessels, resulting in an improved pattern of blood flow....

The brain appears to possess a sensitive shunting mechanism which routinely "diverts blood from inactive parts of the brain towards the areas stimulated." Should this switch become sluggish, the brain will begin working at less than peak efficiency. "But if one is using the head-down position regularly once or twice a day, then the mechanism is 'set' by the temporary effects of the headstand for optimal concentration during the ensuing few hours on mental tasks."

3. Heart rate is reduced.

Within the carotid artery of the neck is a "baroreceptor," sensitive to arterial blood pressure.

Now this pressure receptor follows the usual physiological pattern of the body in trying to return to normal some function which has become abnormal. So when in the headstand position blood pressure has risen by 20%, this pressure body is stimulated and sends signals to the brain to try to reduce the blood pressure. This can be effected either by slowing of the heart, or by dilation of blood vessels to drain blood away from the neck. Both these effects have been recorded, and in the headstand, blood vessels especially in certain muscles, open to drain away blood. However the significant factor is the fall in pulse rate (from 80/min to 65/min are typical figures). Even rising from a chair and walking round a room will raise the pulse by perhaps 10 beats/min., yet here is a light-to-moderate exercise that actually *reduces* the pulse rate. This is true of nearly any head-down position in Yoga where the carotid body is stimulated, since when the head goes below the heart blood tends to flood into the neck, stimulating the baroreceptor there which will tend to slow the heart.

4. Sleep rhythms are normalized.

Wakefulness is maintained as long as the cerebral cortex is bombarded by nerve impulses from the reticular formation.

Now it is found that stimulation of the baroreceptor in the neck dulls the reticular formation and calms it down. Thus the headstand promotes an improved pattern of blood flow through the brain, but at the same time quietens down the reticular formation. Practice of headstand does not make people sleepy; but there are many claims that practiced before going to bed, it helps cure insomnia, and this seems to be the reason.

5. Muscles are efficiently exercised.

The head-down position is also a good exercise as it makes us contract at the same time, opposing sets of muscles by voluntary effort (initiated by the cortex of the brain). The usual way of exercising a muscle is by bending a joint: one muscle is contracted and a reflex arc through the spinal cord relaxes its antagonist. As soon as a message is sent to contract one muscle, another is automatically sent to relax the opposing muscle so that the joint can move. However we sometimes need to contract both sets of muscles to turn the trunk or limb into a solid column, to support ourselves for example. Thus if we consider the headstand position, to prevent the legs collapsing at the knee or hip and to prevent the back from collapsing in various possible ways, agonist and antagonist muscles on both sides of the body must be kept in mild contraction to convert one's body into a pillar that will be able to remain vertical. The arms are of course an exception as one is using them as a support but bent, and not as straight, rigid columns. However elsewhere many muscles are exercised in pairs, so this form of exercise may be considered efficient in this sense.

Further, with the reduction of blood flow to the legs, the active muscles of the back, abdomen, and arms are more generously supplied with blood.

Based on the relatively modest increase in oxygen consumption, Headstand can be classed as a light-to-moderate exercise. According to Dr. Chandra, Headstand, like other light-to-moderate exercise, "burns up fat. Thus it may help you to stay slim) even if it will not actually make you slim)."

Of course Headstand is by no means the only isometric and light-to-moderate exercise in Yoga—almost all static asanas would qualify. But Headstand is unique in not elevating the pulse or speeding up the breath.

6. Pressure in the abdomen is relieved.

Ordinary sitting and standing posture subjects the organs of the abdomen to considerable pressure. The intestines may get blocked and the viscera may be squeezed forward and downward out of position. Tension may accumulate in the supporting muscles. By contrast, Headstand gently stretches the abdominal wall and substantially reduces internal pressure on the organs. Sensations of heaviness or tightness may thus be lessened.

7. Physical imbalances are revealed.

No human body develops in perfect symmetry. But the body adapts so readily to structural anomalies that we are rarely conscious of any process of compensation—at least in the postures we are habituated to. However in inverted postures like Headstand established mechanisms of compensation may not operate. In trying to balance your body weight you may discover areas of comparative stiffness or weakness of which you were not previously aware. Even an unsuccessful attempt to go into Headstand will tell you much about the condition of your body.

CONTRAINDICATIONS

The advantages of Headstand are impressive, but they only accrue to persons practicing it correctly. Practiced incorrectly it may do more harm than good. *Please exercise prudence.* The fact that you *can* do Headstand is not sufficient guarantee that you *ought* to be doing it. Even if you adhere to the fail-safe method given above, it is still conceivable that, for one or another reason, you should not be doing Headstand at all.

We have divided the contraindications into three categories: those which absolutely rule out Headstand, those which make it contingent on a physician's OK, and those which make it merely temporarily inadvisable.

A. Avoid Headstand altogether:

• 1. If you have high blood pressure.

At blood pressures much above normal, the mechanism of "auto-regulation which safeguards the brain from surges of blood... becomes doubtful. If it should fail completely, when one went into the headstand position blood would rush into the brain. This might not do damage at all, however there could be a weak blood vessel somewhere."

Although in the long run the practice of Yoga may help to reduce high blood pressure, it does not follow that all Yoga asanas will be beneficial. You may reasonably aspire to do Headstand even if you presently suffer from high blood pressure (hypertension), but you should not begin practicing it until the pressure has first been brought within normal limits. Other asanas may be of more immediate value.

• 2. If you have ever suffered a concussion.

The effects of a concussion may be latent for years after recovery appears complete. Why take chances?

• 3. If you have a tendency for detachment of the retina—or are extremely shortsighted.

"Although the brain itself has a protective mechanism to prevent an in-rush of blood, the outside of the head and perhaps the retinal veins of the eye may not. Any tendency for detachment of the retina may possibly be aggravated by the head-down position therefore." (Dr. Chandra)

• 4. If you have a history of deafness, vertigo, or chronic ear infection.

Hearing problems are not in themselves a contraindication for Headstand, but they suggest the possibility of malfunction in the vestibular system—responsible for orientation and balance—which is also located in the ear. Even if you have only a mild aversion to being upside down you should avoid Headstand temporarily. Practicing Shoulderstand will gradually accustom you to the sensation of being inverted, but without fear of toppling.

• 5. During pregnancy:

    a) with a tendency to abort.
    b) after the third month, in any case.

Headstand may even help if only temporarily, to bring a retroverted womb out of the pelvis....After three months however the womb is out of the pelvis and one should phase out headstand. The centre of gravity is changing as the weight increases and this will also make it difficult to balance. There are still many useful exercises one can use; breathing, back strengthening, perineal stretching and so on. One does not need to stop practicing Yoga during pregnancy, one simply changes the pattern of practice.

B. Practice Headstand only with the permission of your physician:

- 1. If you are over 40.
- 2. If you are overweight.
- 3. If you have a heart condition.
- 4. If you have low blood pressure.
- 5. If you have a history of surgery or serious disease.
- 6. If you suffer from chronic back, joint, or neck pain.
- 7. If you have frequent headaches.
- 8. If you have chronic sinus trouble.
- 9. If you have become pregnant.

C. In addition, the following may be thought of as temporary contraindications.

Although you may be very experienced, it would not be advisable to practice Headstand:

- 1. If you haven't prepared it with other asanas, or will have no time afterward for adequate compensation. The preparation and counterpose for Headstand are essential, and will be discussed shortly.

- 2. If you cannot do any one of the prerequisite asanas. These will be listed in the next section.

- 3. If you cannot do Headstand according to the technique described earlier. There are other ways of standing on your head (making a tripod of head and hands instead of head and elbows, for example), but these entail additional risk. First, be sure you can do Headstand easily using the ten-step method advocated here.

PREREQUISITES

Assuming Headstand is not contraindicated for reasons of health or circumstance, anyone at all may practice it. Just be sure you are able to do all of the following:

1. Supine Rest

You should be comfortable lying flat on the mat without needing a pillow under your head. If in this position you occasionally experience dizziness or have difficulty breathing through the nose, these symptoms will be exaggerated in Headstand.

2. Floor-Touch (See page 51.)

The forward-bending movements test your readiness to stay in the head-down position. If while doing Floor-Touch you cannot breathe easily through the nose, or feel alternately heavy and light in the head, you should not attempt Headstand.

3. Pyramid (See page 57.)

Pyramid accustoms the head to hanging downward, and prepares the arms, shoulders, and back for bearing weight.

4. Shoulderstand (See page 68.)

You must be able to remain in Shoulderstand with controlled breathing, since this is the prime counterpose for Headstand. It is also an excellent index of the body's readiness to accept the more extreme inverted posture.

5. Plough (See pages 71-72.)

If you cannot easily lift and lower the legs in Plough, your back is not yet strong enough to bear the weight of your legs in Headstand. And if you cannot interlock the fingers with arms stretched on the mat, your shoulders may be too stiff for Headstand.

6. Cobra (See pages 65-66.)

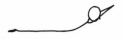

7. Arc (See pages 67-68.)

Both of these test the overall strength of the back muscles, and are typical counterposes for Shoulderstand. The longer you stay in Headstand, the longer you will need to stay in Shoulderstand. The latter too will need compensation, so you should already be proficient in Cobra and Arc.

If you can do these seven asanas you can practice Headstand. Preparation and caution are still essential, so we shall reiterate the basic points we have made about them.

PREPARATION

1. Limber up with a few minutes of easy bending/stretching movements, either standing, kneeling, sitting, or supine. These should answer the questions:

   •How is my breath?
   •How is my body, in general?
   •How is my neck, in particular?
   •Shall I proceed with Headstand?

2. Lie on the back and rest for a minute or more.

PRECAUTIONS

1. Be sure your pad is thick enough.
2. Practice against a wall until you are absolutely confident you can dispense with it.
3. Go into Headstand by easy stages.
4. Press the elbows and keep the legs slightly bent, for optimum balance and control.

5. Breathe deeply at all times.
6. Come down slowly.

COMPENSATIONS

First of all, rest on your back for a minute or more.

Then, optionally, you may do a few breaths of Bridge (dynamically) and/or Knee Hold. (See pages 45, 46 and 47.)

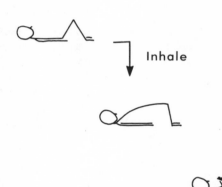

Inhale

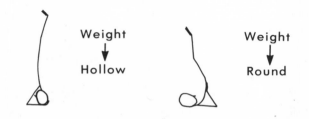

Weight → Hollow

Weight → Round

Weight borne by hollow back and neck.

Weight borne by round back and neck.

Shoulderstand should be maintained for at least as many breaths as Headstand, to have the full effect. It is not mandatory (as with other counterposes) to do dynamic variations, since the isometric stress in Shoulderstand perfectly complements that in Headstand. However, leg-lowering movements can be advantageous. (See pages 68-72.)

Integrating inverted poses into your Yoga practice will be further discussed in Chapter 9.

The recommended counterpose for Headstand is Shoulderstand, since it, among other things:

1. Stretches the muscles at the back of the neck.
2. Contracts the fore muscles of the neck.
3. Rounds the back.
4. Stretches the spinal muscles.
5. Uses the weight of the legs to make the back work in a way opposite and almost equal to Headstand.
6. Allows you to prolong the benefits of being inverted.

8

ELEMENTS OF PRANAYAMA

Pranayama is the culmination of asana. As any posture becomes more stable and comfortable you can devote increasing attention to the breath. Asanas are the ideal preparation for pranayama. Not only do they limber and strengthen the body to the point where extended sitting is easy, but they help you develop better breathing habits along with added control. Just as pranayama evolves from the practice of asanas over a period of time, so in each practice session should pranayama come after a course of asanas. It is important to understand that asana and pranayama are essentially indivisible; they are but the two ends of a continuum. Every asana is in part pranayama, and no pranayama can exist without asana.

ASANA IN PRANAYAMA

Of course asanas are not all equally suitable for practicing pranayama. In Chapter 4 we mentioned some of the more useful ones. The simplest is Supine Rest (*Shavāsana*). It is the best one for beginners and it is also the pose of choice when you are tired—no matter how advanced you are in Yoga. In Supine Rest there is no effort required to maintain an erect carriage; you can apply your energy entirely to breathing. Later in this chapter we will indicate what kind of pranayama is feasible in Supine Rest.

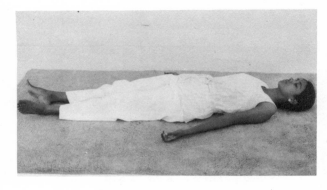

Supine Rest

You may also sit on a chair or bench—one which is not too soft, and which supports your thighs while the feet rest on the floor. Use as little back support as necessary—ideally, none at all. Spread the legs for added comfort.

Another feasible pose is Kneeling Seat (*Vajrāsana*). It allows you to keep the trunk erect with little effort, but can put quite a strain on the ankles and kneecaps. The latter are particularly vulnerable to injury, so be careful. If you are comfortable sitting in this pose you may use it for your pranayama, especially if stiff hips and tight muscles along the inside of the legs make cross-legged sitting difficult.

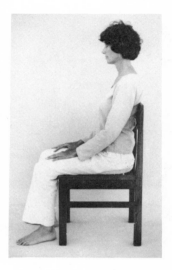

Chair Seat   or

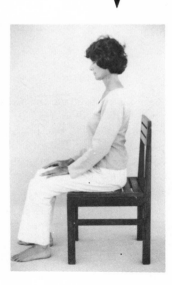

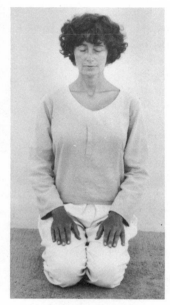

Kneeling Seat

Cross-Legged Seat (*Sukhāsana*) lets you sit straight without too much effort and does not require exceptional flexibility in the hips and legs. Thus it is a good compromise pose for pranayama. As suggested in Chapter 4, a cushion under the buttocks will simplify Cross-Legged Seat, until your back muscles become strong and thighs loosen up.

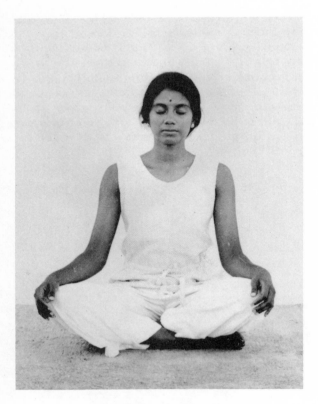

Cross-Legged Seat

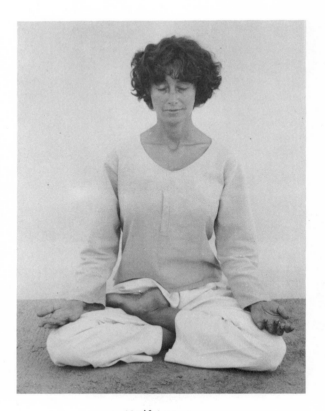

Half Lotus

Those who are more supple may prefer to sit in Half Lotus (*Ardha Padmāsana*). One bent leg rests on the mat while the other leg, similarly bent, rests atop the first: thigh on foot and foot on thigh. Since Half Lotus is not entirely symmetrical, it would be advisable, if you use it regularly, to alternate the legs: one day right above left, and the next day left above right.

More extreme and better known is the full Lotus (*Padmasana*). It is a posture of great beauty and poise. Legs are bent, thighs on the mat, and feet placed one by one on opposite thighs. Provided your legs are up to it, you can hold the back erect with hardly any effort. However, unless you have been practicing Lotus for years, you will likely experience considerable pressure on the shins and loss of blood circulation to the feet. Afterward you may feel sore around the joints—hips, knees, and ankles—if your leg muscles are at all stiff.

If you are keen on mastering Lotus, a good teacher can suggest some preparatory exercises which you can incorporate in your asana practice. Please note that the Model Practice Sequence in Chapter 3 was not designed with any such specialized intent; however attractive, Lotus need not be a basic fitness objective for most people.

If you do sit in Lotus for pranayama, you might observe the suggestion made above regarding alternating the legs in successive practices. Lotus appears quite symmetrical but in fact there is more of a pull around that hip whose knee is the higher.

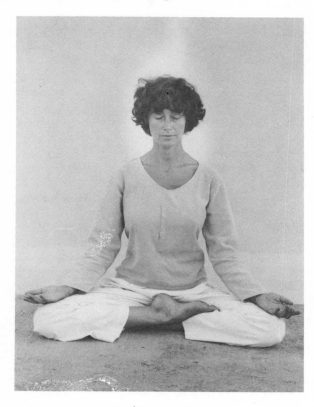

Lotus

Meditation Seat

Less sensational but equally harmonious is Meditation Seat (*Siddhāsana*). Like the full and half Lotus it is advantageous to the back, but without hampering circulation in the calves. Meditation Seat is almost perfectly symmetrical. Both legs rest on the mat, with one heel—let us say the left—wedged against the perineum (the soft place between the thighs) and the right heel drawn up unto the left foot, close to the left heel. As in Cross-Legged Seat, you may be able to increase your staying power by pulling a cushion underneath you.

However you choose to sit for pranayama, try to hold your back straight, in order to permit optimum expansion of the thorax. Lowering the chin slightly will help to keep your neck relaxed. Close your eyes during pranayama; let them rest for a while. Arms should hang loosely, without tension in the shoulders.

If you like, you may rest the back of each hand on its thigh, near the knee. This facilitates counting the breaths on the fingers. The thumb serves as counter, and advances to each finger segment in a clockwise spiral (if you are using the left hand):

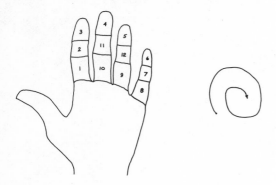

The tip of the little finger, for example, always represents "6"; when the thumb reaches it you know you have completed 6 breaths. If you don't want to be bothered counting in this way you may rest your palms on your thighs or place your hands in your lap.

THE FOUR-PHASE CYCLE

Up till now we have been assuming that there are only two parts to the breath—in and out—however much we may deepen and extend them. For all ordinary purposes, and even for asana most of the time, the assumption holds. What chiefly distinguishes pranayama is not so much its repertory of techniques as the importance it gives to the *intervals* possible between the active movements of respiration. A full exhalation followed by a full inhalation certainly qualifies as a "complete breath," but even a complete breath can be extended by holds.

Pranayama posits an expanded, four-phase breath cycle, consisting of:

Inhalation	(*Pūraka*)
Retention	(*Antah kumbhaka*)
Exhalation	(*Rechaka*)
Suspension	(*Bāhya kumbhaka*)

What we have termed retention and suspension can as well be called "holding the breath *in*" and "holding the breath *out*." *Kumbhaka* means "pot-like"; *antaḥ* and *bāhya* are "inner" and "outer," respectively. (The metaphor can easily be conjectured.) *Pūraka* literally means "filling up," and *rechaka* means "emptying."

Although pranayama admits a maximum of four phases it by no means requires the presence of all four. You need not hold the breath at all (beyond pausing for a moment, as in asanas, to separate inhalation from exhalation, and vice versa). Or you can decide to hold the breath after *either* inhalation or exhalation. Here, each complete breath cycle would comprise not just the fundamental two phases, inhaling and exhaling, but a third— holding. Suspension without retention is effective in certain cases. Retention without suspension is a more usual pattern, for a good reason. Exhalation is typically longer than inhalation and is easier to control. Holding after inhalation thus helps to balance the breath timewise, and to increase one's control over the action of inhalation. If you want to include both retention *and* suspension you will have to reduce their length accordingly.

In short, we have these four permutations:

1. Inhalation—Exhalation
2. Inhalation—Retention—Exhalation
3. Inhalation—Exhalation—Suspension
4. Inhalation—Retention—Exhalation— Suspension

We shall soon see how these intersect with some of the more common techniques of pranayama.

As can be inferred from the following graphs, holding the breath both prolongs and intensifies the effect of in- and exhalation.

1. Inhalation—Exhalation

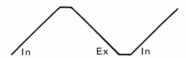

2. Inhalation—Retention—Exhalation

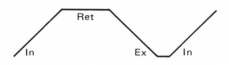

3. Inhalation—Exhalation—Suspension

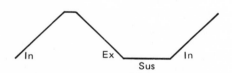

4. Inhalation—Retention—Exhalation Suspension

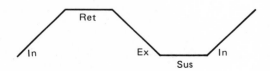

The longer the hold, the stronger the effect:

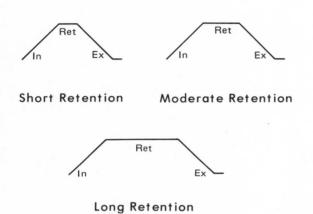

Short Retention   Moderate Retention

Long Retention

You will discover also that holding the breath impinges on the *length* of inhalation or exhalation; there is a time limit to your maximum breath cycle. A long hold after inhalation, for example, may deduct time from the following exhalation:

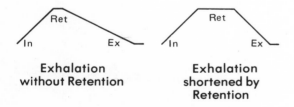

Exhalation   Exhalation
without Retention   shortened by
    Retention

How you choose to utilize breath holding depends on your reason for doing pranayama. In general, you would use some retention if your inhalation needs extending, and suspension if your exhalation is too quick. We shall elaborate this principle somewhat, but in a book of this scope it will not be possible to explain all the nuances of pranayama.

If you decide to experiment in your pranayama with some holding of the breath, try to go about it in the same progressive spirit with which you learned the Model Practice Sequence. Start with a very modest retention, say 4-5 seconds, for the first few days. And even when you have built up your capacity to 8-10 seconds or longer, you should begin each day's pranayama with little or no holding and gradually increase it by stages.

Breath holding may also be employed to a more limited extent while practicing asanas. Choose an asana which is comfortable for you; do it dynamically a few times, then hold for a few breaths. Now, without speeding up the rate of inhalation or exhalation, see if you can add several seconds of retention after inhalation. Suspension after exhalation may also be useful in certain asanas. Breath holding can increase the therapeutic value of asanas—though in some cases it may be counterproductive. This is yet another area that is difficult to explore without a skilled teacher.

VARIETIES OF PRANAYAMA

For the reader curious to experiment further with pranayama, we shall now describe four basic varieties, with reference to the placement of the breath, the four-phase cycle, and the purposes to which each may be put.

1. Throat-Sound Inhalation—Throat-Sound Exhalation (*Ujjāyī*)

We defined throat-sound breathing in Chapter 6. It is used here for both inhalation and exhalation. This is the only pranayama which may be comfortably practiced supine as well as seated. Although *Ujjāyī* may be the easiest type of pranayama it can also be the most difficult—depending on the relative and absolute durations of inhalation, exhalation, and optional holding. Their absolute length cannot be prescribed in a book, since breath capacity varies so much from person to person. What is trivial for one person will be very arduous for another. Therefore, the only numbers which are to be taken in an exact sense in the following discussions are those referring to the *relative* length of the four phases - what we shall be calling the *ratio* of the breath. Every ratio is possible for every person, so long as you select absolute values that are modest enough.

The Seated Breathing which concluded the Model Practice Sequence is one typical example of Ujjayi. At the time we presented it, in Chapters 3 and 4, it would have been premature to include too much detail on the technique of Yoga breathing, throat sound, etc. We did introduce the term *rechaka* pranayama, or "long-exhalation breathing," so called because the rechaka, or exhalation, phase is deliberately prolonged. The long exhalation may be free (as in Chapter 3, Course #1) or measured. The standard ratio for long-exhalation breathing (suggested in Course #3) is 1:2—which is short for 1:0:2:0. As explained in the instructions, your inhalation should be only long enough that you can make the exhalation last twice as long. In terms of seconds, this ratio would be as validly expressed by 3.6 as by 6.12. Whether you choose seconds or some other counting unit, the beats must be regular. A metronome or other timing device may be of assistance. To repeat, it is not the ratio that makes a pranayama

difficult, but absolute values that are too ambitious.

Ujjayi lends itself well to the ratio 1:2, which is a very soothing one. Long exhalations, in particular, appear to activate the parasympathetic nervous system—the so-called "relaxation response." Another classic ratio for Ujjayi is 1:1, i.e., equal inhalation and exhalation, as for example 4.4 or 8.8. Still other proportions are possible. If you can do 6.6 but not 6.12, you might try 6.9, which would represent the intermediate ratio 1:1½.

Holding the breath can be quite useful in Ujjayi. Suppose you have mastered 6.12 (1:0:2:0) or 8.8 (1:0:1:0). An excellent way of progressing toward longer breaths is simply to add a little retention. From 6.12 you might advance by stages to 6.3.12 (1:½:2:0) and then to 6.6.12 (1:1:2:0). In the other example, you could intensify 8.8 with graded retention: 8.4.8 (1:½:1:0), then 8.8.8 (1:1:1:0:). Since the exhalation is not long with respect to inhalation, it would be possible to add some suspension as well: e.g., 8.4.8.4 (1:½:1:½) or 8.8.8.4 (1:1:1:½). When you get used to holding the breath, you have always the option of stepping up your basic unit. If you master 8.8.8, for example, why not try 10.0.10? And so on.

2. Throat-Sound Inhalation—Alternate-Nostril Exhalation (*Anuloma Ujjāyī*)

In *Anuloma Ujjāyī* it is only on inhalation that we place the breath in the throat. On exhalation, in order to make the breath slower still, we employ a special technique of pranayama known as "single-nostril," or "alternate-nostril," breathing. Here only one nostril at a time is left open, and even it is partially depressed by one or more fingers, acting as a valve, to reduce the diameter of the nasal passage at will.

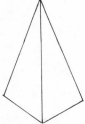

Throat sound

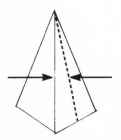

Single Nostril

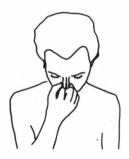

Breathing through
left or right nostril

Obviously, this technique must be used with discretion, since you are physically obstructing the normal flow of the breath. Never use force to restrain the breath, lest you experience pressure and pain in the head. Sensibly practiced, however, single-nostril breathing helps to strengthen the muscles of the abdomen and chest which control the breath, and leads gradually to greater control even when both nostrils are wide open (i.e., in throat-sound breathing).

As customarily practiced, single-nostril breathing utilizes the right hand exclusively. The upper arm is held loosely at the side, bent at the elbow. The thumb is used to depress the right nostril, and the ring and little fingers together depress the left nostril. The index and middle fingers, which are not needed, are curled toward the palm. When you want to breathe through the left nostril (whether in or out), you close off the right nostril completely with the thumb, pressing just where the nasal bone ends. Fourth and fifth fingers press *gently* against the left nostril, regulating the aperture as desired. To breathe through the right nostril, reverse the pressure of thumb and fingers.

The head should remain centered; try not to turn or tilt it to left or right as you press against the nose. Note that single-nostril pranayama is practicable only in a seated posture. If you try it in Supine Rest your right arm may tire too quickly for you to continue very long.

If your nostrils are clogged you will experience some discomfort in this pranayama, since you will not be able to get all the stale air out in time to take a fresh breath. In this case, throat Ujjayi would be a better choice. But if one or both nostrils are only slightly congested, Anuloma Ujjayi may help to clear them.

We have talked of asymmetry with regard to asanas; Anuloma Ujjayi is an example of an "asymmetrical" pranayama. After inhaling (with throat sound) through both nostrils, you raise the forearm, place the fingers over the bridge of the nose, as described, and begin to exhale through one (partially squeezed) nostril. Having inhaled again through the throat, exhale through the other nostril. It doesn't matter whether your first exhalation passed through the left or right nostril; but having begun, maintain the same alternating pattern.

Should you discover, in practicing throat Ujjayi, that you lack control over exhalation, relative to inhalation, you might try the same ratio with single-nostril exhalations. The reduced diameter of the nasal passage will slow down the rate at which the air escapes, giving you extra time to feel your abdominal muscles contracting. This controlled abdominal underpinning to the gradual release of the breath is what actors, singers, and wind instrument players call "supporting the breath," or "diaphragmatic breathing." However you visualize it, Anuloma Ujjayi is a good way to practice it. As you get accustomed to using your abdominal muscles you will find your exhalations lengthening even when both nostrils are open.

Anuloma Ujjayi has a further advantage. Exhalation is always easier to regulate through one nostril than through the throat, regardless of ratio. The facility it gives allows you to take more liberty with inhalation and retention. Taking 1:0:2, for example, you may be able to use a larger unit value than was possible in throat Ujjayi. Or you can experiment with retention, in ratios like 1:½:2, 1:1:2, 1:1½:2, 1:2:2, 1:3:2, or even 1:4:2. When you are used to retention in Anuloma Ujjayi, you might also incorporate some suspension. Again taking 1:2 as a basis, you could try 1:½:2:½, 1:1:2:½, 1:1:2:1, 1:2:2:1, 1:4:2:1.

Does the mathematics of pranayama put you off? Rest easy: pranayama was never intended to be learned from books. (How much will the study of grammar improve your fluency in a spoken language?) You really need a teacher to suggest suitable breathing exercises for you and to keep track of your progress.

3. Alternate-Nostril Inhalation—Throat-Sound Exhalation (Viloma Ujjāyī)

This pranayama will aid you in developing more control over inhalation—provided that is really

what you need. It assumes that you have no difficulty prolonging exhalation.

Inhale with finger pressure, through left and right nostrils alternately, exhaling each time as in throat Ujjayi. Since the object is to increase inhalation at the expense of (a disproportionately long) exhalation, you would normally avoid ratios like 1:2. Since inhalation time should never exceed exhalation, you should avoid theoretical ratios like 2:1. Instead, stay close to the standard 1:1, as described under Ujjayi.

If a 1:1 throat inhalation with seemingly modest values is taxing, and you are finishing the inhalations too soon, you might have more success with Viloma Ujjayi. Inhaling through only one nostril, with adjustable finger pressure, may be easier; it certainly gives you more chance to practice control. If you are getting somewhere with this pranayama and need to increase the challenge, add some retention: e.g., 1:½:1 or 1:1:1. The next step would be to increase the absolute values: e.g., in progressive order, 8.0.8, 8.4.8, 8.8.8; 10.0.10, 10.5.10, etc.

Note: If your nostrils are congested you should not do Viloma Ujjayi or the pranayama described next.

4. Alternate-Nostril Inhalation and Exhalation (Nāḍishodhana)

If you have been practicing the several types of Ujjayi you may also try Nāḍishodhana, in which both inhalation and exhalation are made through one nostril. A complete cycle, comprising two breaths, has the sequence:

Inhale: left nostril — Exhale: right nostril
Inhale: right nostril — Exhale: left nostril

Since you can voluntarily regulate both halves of the breath, Nadishodhana gives you the most scope for prolonging total breath span of any pranayama we have discussed. The same ratios you have been using in throat Ujjayi and Anuloma Ujjayi may be practiced in Nadishodhana. In some cases larger absolute values may be possible. If 8.8 was comfortable for you in throat breathing, you may find single-nostril 10.10, or even 12.12, no more demanding. Retention and suspension may also enter the picture. In addition to the ratios listed so far, Nadishodhana lends itself to such as the following: 2:1:2:0 ($=1:\frac{1}{2}:1:0$), 2:1:2:1, 2:2:2:0, 2:2:2:1, 3:1:3:0, 3:2:3:0, 3:1:3:1, 3:3:3:0, 2:1:4:0, 2:1:4:1, 2:2:4:0, 2:2:4:1, etc.

One disadvantage of Nadishodhana is that it requires that your hand be raised to the nose for long periods. Your right arm may get tired after a while.

ADDITIONAL VARIETIES

For the record, here are thumbnail sketches of some further varieties of pranayama. They presuppose considerable familiarity with the four we have just discussed, and it would be pointless to practice them without a teacher's guidance.

1. Pratiloma Ujjāyī

This is a combination of Anuloma and Viloma Ujjayi. A single cycle takes four breaths:

Inhale: throat	— Exhale: L nostril
Inhale: L nostril	— Exhale: throat
Inhale: throat	— Exhale: R nostril
Inhale: R nostril	— Exhale: throat

Different ratios and holding are possible, as in Ujjayi.

2. Sūryabhedana and Chandrabhedana

These are strictly asymmetrical pranayamas. *Sūryabhedana* is useful in unblocking the left nostril:

Inhale: R nostril — Exhale: L nostril
Inhale: R nostril — Exhale: L nostril (and so on)

Chandrabhedana is the reverse: all inhalations through the left nostril, all exhalations through the right.

3. Anuloma, Viloma, and Pratiloma Krama

These are techniques of interrupted breathing, used by advanced practitioners to further deepen control and maintain attention. In *Anuloma Krama*, you inhale for several seconds, hold the breath several seconds, inhale some more, hold some more, etc. Exhalation is straightforward, either with throat sound or through alternate nostrils. In *Viloma Krama* it is the exhalation which is interrupted; and in *Pratiloma* both inhalation and exhalation. Interrupted breathing may be used with any of the pranayamas so far discussed.

Here are some examples:

Anuloma Krama: Inhale 5, hold 5, inhale 5, hold 5; exhale 10.
Viloma Krama: Inhale 10, exhale 5, hold 5, exhale 5, hold 5.
Pratiloma Krama: Inhale 4, hold 4, inhale 4, hold 4; exhale 4, hold 4, exhale 4, hold 4.

4. Shītalī

In this unique and useful pranayama you inhale not through the nose at all, but through the mouth—by curling the tongue between the lips to form a sort of duct. After each inhalation the tongue is drawn in and rolled upward toward the palate. Exhalation can be made either with throat sound or through alternate nostrils, as desired.

5. Kapālabhāti and Bhastrikā

These two are sometimes employed to clear the respiratory tract, exchange stale air in the lungs for fresh, and to quickly warm up the chest.

Kapālabhāti is a rapid breathing, with rhythmical abdominal contractions. Suck in the abdomen as you exhale; let it relax outward as the air is drawn in.

Bhastrikā ("bellows") is similar, but is specific for clearing the nose. Inhale and exhale rapidly through the same nostril or through alternate nostrils (as in Nadishodhana).

Be careful not to overdo these two. Forceful contractions should be avoided unless your abdominal muscles are already well developed, and should never be practiced during pregnancy, or if you have a urogenital condition, a hernia, etc. Fast breathing may make you dizzy. It is advisable to include several rounds of slow breathing at regular intervals; for example, 16 breaths fast, 4 slow; 16 fast, 4 slow.

6. The Bandhas

The *bandhas* are special muscular contractions sometimes used in pranayama (and in certain asanas). They are possible only when the back is straight. There are three bandhas and they work together. The first, a chin lock, and the second, a contraction at the base of the abdomen, can be retained throughout the breath cycle. The third bandha is an inward and upward suction of the abdomen which is possible only after exhalation has been completed, and which must be relaxed prior to inhaling again. The bandhas are not for everyone. They should be practiced only under the guidance of a teacher.

PRACTICING PRANAYAMA

When it comes to pranayama, misconceptions abound, even among those who have already been introduced to Yoga practice. Many people are overawed by pranayama and assume it is beyond their level of attainment. Others are skeptical about "interfering" in any way with the breath. Some see pranayama as a purely symbolic gesture whose purpose is served by a couple of perfunctory breaths. Active, sociable people are often embarrassed to sit by themselves and breathe, finding it a waste of valuable time—if not downright sinful! Even some practitioners of Yoga feel the time would better be spent doing a few additional asanas. Or else they so exhaust themselves doing asanas that they lack the energy to do anything afterward but rest or sleep. At the other extreme are those who, thinking that pranayama represents a higher stage of Yoga than mere asanas, try to short-circuit the process and eliminate asanas altogether.

We have sought to establish that pranayama is an integral part of Yoga practice, that it is essentially inseparable from asana, that it should be prepared by at least a short course of asanas, and that it can be practiced to advantage by anyone.

The ratios, techniques, and varieties we have described are not so much the substance of pranayama as its instruments. Their function is to insure that involvement with the breath is always fresh. Start with basic varieties, simple ratios, and modest time values. Add only enough complexity to maintain interest and perhaps a slight challenge.

Pranayama requires patience and intelligence. Don't try to lengthen your breath all of a sudden or to hold your breath for exaggerated intervals. Be guided by this precept from the *Hatha Yoga Pradīpikā* (II.15): "As lions, elephants, and tigers may be tamed, so also the prana may be controlled: gradually, lest it cause harm."

We have gone to some length to explain why breath is essential to Yoga. By way of conclusion, we may summarize as follows:

1. Good breathing promotes physical health and well-being. It particularly benefits the heart and lungs.

2. Yoga breathing can be deeply relaxing. It increases vitality and calms the mind.

3. Observing the breath in asana and especially in pranayama is an easy way of centering—a tangible kind of meditation.

9

COMPOSING YOUR OWN COURSE

Throughout this book we have been emphasizing that Yoga can and must be adapted to the needs of individuals. So by now you are probably wondering how Yoga can be of most use to *you*. Which asanas should *you* practice? In what way? Which types of pranayama make most sense? No book can do justice to these very legitimate questions. For that you must have a competent teacher who knows you well. However, we can at least suggest some basic guidelines (recapitulating and amplifying where necessary) to give you a fair idea how you personally can derive maximum benefit from the practice of Yoga.

TIME

The first factor to consider in composing your own course is *time*. There is no sense in planning an elaborate course if you have only a few minutes in which to execute it. Ideally, time should be at the service of Yoga, but we all know that real-world pressures make this impossible. You will almost always know how much time you can afford to spend on Yoga, so it makes good sense to take that into consideration before you get started.

Relating also to time is the question "When?". A course that works for you in the evening may not be appropriate for a morning practice. One that

works in the summer may not work in winter. One that feels good when you are well may not when you are ill. Conversely, a course designed for a special problem or condition may be pointless when you are fit and healthy. A practice which is effective when you are new to Yoga may not be satisfying after you have become more adept. A course which is feasible when you are young may become less so as you grow older.

ORGANIZATION AND ECONOMY

Depending on the time available you can determine the basic organization of your course. If your time is limited and you want to exercise the body, do a group of asanas and rest. If your time is limited and you want to concentrate on breathing, do some pranayama and rest. Since you will probably not have time for all the Yoga exercises you know or enjoy doing, you will have to select some of them and leave out others. Just be sure to allow ample time for resting—the importance of which was emphasized in Chapter 4.[1]

Theoretically you could spend a great deal of time on a great many asanas, in order to be sure of having touched on those areas which most need work. And this approach might succeed, provided you had sufficient time to spare, didn't get bored easily, and managed not to overtire yourself. But obviously the risk of abandoning the effort altogether would be high. For any Yoga course to be effective it must be practiced frequently. If the course is too long or too ambitious it will be often postponed, if not entirely abandoned. Hence the very practical constraint of *economy*. The course should be no longer than the time realistically available, and it should be limited in its objectives.

The structure and character of your course largely depend on your objective, whether it be to mitigate a particular condition or merely to improve general fitness. But some features of the course are always valid: it must have an adequate *prelude*, and it must include sufficient *preparation* and *compensation* for all but the simplest asanas.

PRELUDE

The first step in any course of asanas is to *discover the status of the body*; the second is to *ready the body* for physical demands. As it happens, both can be accomplished together, by means of easy stretching and bending movements.

As long as your body is inert, you cannot know what condition the limbs and organs are in. But a little movement will quickly tell you. This is particularly important if you are beginning your Yoga practice after sleep or several hours of sitting. Most likely you will discover nothing amiss, but in case you do find an unexpected stiffness or tenderness it is well that you know of it before launching into more demanding asanas. You still have ample time to reorient your course accordingly.

It is also useful, at the outset, to observe the condition of the breath. If your breathing is still erratic after several rounds of preliminary stretching, you can amend your course to work on the part of the breath that is weak.

Readying the body for physical demands is the aim of warming up. If you have been inactive for some time beforehand, circulation in your limbs and joints will have diminished. The colder the air outside the body, the greater the tendency for constriction of the superficial and outlying blood vessels, in order that the blood and body heat be concentrated near the vital organs of the head and trunk. If you plan on exercising the muscles and joints, particularly in the limbs, you must therefore make a point of inducing blood flow to these areas.

The best way of accomplishing both objectives is generally through standing asanas.[2] However, if you are already warm, or if you have been on your feet for some time, or if your legs feel heavy, you may substitute some kneeling or sitting movements. If you are especially tired, you can begin by doing some breathing on your back.

The prelude should take 5-10 minutes, and may include one or more asanas. These should be done slowly and with attention to the breath. In between the movements you may want either to take one or more free breaths, or to hold the breath for several seconds. The safest movements to begin with are arm raising or forward-bending. Side stretching and twisting may then be introduced, if you like. Backbending poses, however, are better postponed until you are already warmed up.

Although the prelude is essential at the beginning of any course, it need not become stale or ritualized. There are an infinite number of ways to warm up and investigate the body. These cannot be standardized since no two individuals are alike, and no one individual is the same at all times. But using the Model Practice Sequence as a guide and drawing upon the asanas in Chapter 5, you should be able to construct any number of excellent warm-up sequences.

The prelude is best completed by resting for a short while on the back. It is thus set apart from the main body of the course.

PREPARATION

Just as the prelude serves to prepare you for the more demanding phase of the course, so the effect of each prominent asana is enhanced by prior preparation. To "prepare" an asana, you must first predict or recollect how it will work on your body. Then select one or more asanas having a similar effect, but which are milder. These asanas should be done before the one toward which they aim, and should be performed rather more dynamically than statically.

Thus, if the object of a hypothetical course is to stay 8 breaths in Arc, it would make sense to have done some Swimmer and/or Cobra beforehand, with an emphasis on repetition rather than staying:

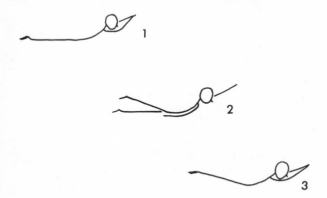

Ordinarily, the preparatory asanas should each be followed by an appropriate relaxing asana. In this way a logical course structure begins to evolve.

To take another example, suppose you want to sit in Volcano for 12 long breaths on each side:

This is a feasible objective, but it may be too strenuous without sufficient preparation. The immediate precursor might be some dynamic stretching in a similarly seated position, such as Sitting Stretch or One-Leg Stretch:

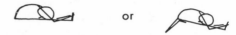

The seated stretching, too, may be prepared in the prelude by some standing or kneeling forward-bending, e.,g., Floor-Touch, Striding Stretch, Kneeling Bend, or the equivalent:

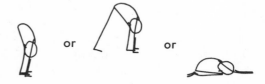

While on your back after the prelude, you might rest the back in Knee Hold and prepare the neck with Bridge:

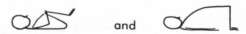

Having prepared the body in this fashion, you will get more out of Volcano, with much less chance of negative side-effects.

COMPENSATION

The rationale for compensation is much the same: to obviate the negative effects of an asana while retaining only the positive.

The fact that we recommend counterposes in Yoga does not mean that Yoga is especially dangerous. Every physical activity—or inactivity—exacts a price. Not only sports, but walking, standing, sitting, even lying down can have negative consequences along with the good. Using muscles tends to stiffen the joints. Standing causes blood to accumulate in the legs. Sitting in chairs is bad for the back and encourages flabbiness. Too much resting decreases muscle tone and blood pressure. Thus, unless prevented from doing so, we unconsciously change position frequently.

Ideally we should compensate for all our activities, but it is not always possible to do so when activity is not an end in itself, but is rather at the service of some other motivation. In Yoga, however, where the whole point is to devote full attention to the body and the breath, there is no excuse for not taking minimal precautions. If anything, asanas are *safer* than other physical activities, but in Yoga we have the means to avoid harm altogether.

Hopefully there will be some carry-over from the use of counterposes in Yoga, just as the practice of Yoga breathing may improve the quality of the breath *after* exercise. As you acquire the habit of compensating for postures in Yoga you may become more sensitive to the way you use your body at other times.

Counterposes were built into the Model Practice Sequence; their use was explained in Chapter 4.

One or more counterposes were suggested for each of the asanas in the "Anthology." It remains now merely to abstract the basic principles of compensation so that you can apply them with confidence in your own personalized practice.

1. The asana you use as a compensation will vary according to the effect on you of the previous asana.

In choosing a counterpose for Cobra, for example, you must decide whether it is the neck or the back which most needs it. In the former case, Bridge is indicated; in the latter, Knee Hold:

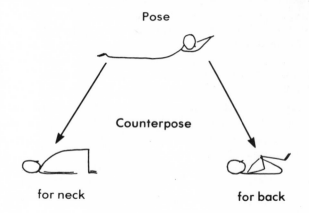

Pose

Counterpose

for neck   for back

Of course, you could do both just to play safe. Multiplied by several more asanas, however, this approach might unnecessarily lengthen the course. In most cases, a single counterpose will do, provided you have correctly understood how the asana is working on your body.

2. The need for compensation is somewhat lessened if the asana has been adequately prepared, and done dynamically before statically. Going right to the final pose is a false economy. You will have to spend that much longer on counter-

poses and they may not be as effective in preventing soreness.

3.   Compensation is advisable even when you feel no immediate need for it, lest there be a delayed side-effect. This applies particularly to backbends, twists, and inverted poses. You may feel nothing while your body is still warm, but the joints and muscles may remain in a state of tension and cause you pain later on.

4.   It is good to rest on the back after certain poses—such as Headstand and Shoulderstand[3]— before beginning the counterpose. When the back and neck have been strongly contracted in one direction it is better not to contract them the other way until they have been allowed to relax. A brief rest after a demanding posture should make you more attentive to the effect of the counterpose.

5.   To be effective, a counterpose must not only counteract the asana; it must be *easier* than the asana. You gain nothing if the compensation is more strenuous than what it is supposed to be compensating.

In Chapter 5 we suggested Squat as a counterpose to Floor-Touch. Quite possibly, Squat may be *more* rather than less difficult (even in a simplified version), in which case you can substitute an easier flexing counterpose, such as Kneeling Bend:

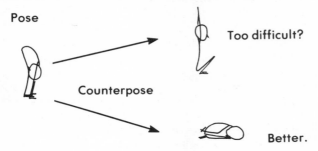

Pose

Too difficult?

Counterpose

Better.

6.   The asana requiring compensation may or may not have been done statically, but the counterpose should ordinarily be done *dynamically*, in order for its effect to be gradual and evenly distributed. Slow movements with breathing accomplish this better than going directly to the final position of the counterpose and remaining still.

7.   Do the counterpose for at least half as many breaths as the asana preceding. Fewer breaths might suffice, but it is better to err on the side of safety.

8.   An asana chosen as counterpose should not itself require a counterpose, lest you get into an unending cycle. (We have already accounted for the special case of Shoulderstand, following Headstand.) You might want to rest after an asana and its counterpose, but you should be free then to continue in any direction.

9.   It stands to reason that before you practice a new asana you should already have learned and become comfortable with its counterpose. Before trying Pyramid, for example, you should be adept at Quadruped.

SYNCHRONOUS BREATHING

We have previously stated the case for synchronous breathing.[4] In composing your own course, along the lines of this book, you should be sure that your asana movements are performed with the correct phase of the breath. As long as you stick to the asanas depicted in Chapters 3 and 5, you need only refer to the breathing directions given in the text. But you may also want to practice asanas not included in this book—and there is no reason why you should not do so. How then should you fit your breathing to the movements?

The breathing directions given for the Model Practice Sequence and the "Anthology of Asanas" are based on two principles which we cited in Chapter 4:

— *Inhale* when executing a movement which naturally encourages the *expansion* of the lungs.

— *Exhale* when the movement encourages *deflation* of the lungs.

In the light of Chapter 6, we can elaborate these rules as follows:

Inhale when the movement:

1) expands the rib cage,
2) hollows the back, or
3) allows the abdomen to relax outward.

Exhale when the movement:

1) compresses the rib cage,
2) rounds the back, or
3) contracts the abdomen.

Instances of *inhalation* movements would be:

1. Raising the arms.
2. Elevating the trunk after a forward bend, or from a prone lying position.
3. Taking the legs away from the chest.
4. Extending the legs from a previously flexed position.
5. Restoring the trunk to a central position after stretching or twisting to one side of the body.
6. Restoring the head or legs to a central position after movement to one side of the body.

Corresponding to these movements and consistent with *exhalation* are:

1. Lowering the arms.
2. Flexing the trunk toward the thighs.
3. Bringing the legs toward the chest.

4. Flexing the legs.
5. Stretching or twisting the trunk to one side of the body.
6. Turning the head or stretching one or both legs to one side of the body.

It should be apparent by now that the connection between breath and body movement is quite scientific. Much of the potential value of Yoga asanas is lost when movement and breath are coordinated haphazardly or not at all.

It may be argued that the notions of prelude, preparation and compensation, and synchronous breathing are not essential to Yoga. Certainly, they are not taught as such in many systems of Yoga instruction. The reason we have emphasized them in this book is that they make it possible for anyone to practice Yoga, with minimum risk and maximum benefit.

PROGRESS

The practice of any discipline soon becomes sterile where a sense of progress is absent. Yoga is no exception. Progress is important psychologically: if you don't feel you are getting anywhere, you are bound to lose interest and slacken your efforts. But the need for progress is more than psychological.

In the process of living we are constantly being confronted by new challenges. The genius of living organisms is their ability to respond. Either the novelty of the challenge is analyzed into more familiar and assimilable constituents, or else the organism itself changes in an effort better to adapt itself to the new demand. Either way there is growth, and as long as there is growth there is life. When an organism ceases to respond to a novel environment it begins to decay. There is rarely a question of "holding your own." Nature has seen to it that you either advance or retreat.

The human body is an organic assembly. It functions as a unit but its members are always in flux. It is superbly equipped to adapt to stress, and is doing so all the time, consciously or not. The purpose of exercising the body is to introduce a deliberate, controlled stress, which is enough to secure adaptive growth but not so much as to cause a breakdown. An exercise which no longer has this effect is no longer an exercise. It must either be intensified, or—if the body has been debilitated—reduced. The idea of "exercising" is anathema to many, but largely because it is not correctly understood. The option of remaining the same is not really granted to us. Like all other life, if we fail to *progress* we *regress*.

If your Yoga practice is to remain fresh you must take advantage of the opportunities for progress. These are, in fact, limitless. In Yoga there is always room for improvement and also the means to achieve it. In working with asanas there are many ways to progress. The most obvious way is to learn new asanas. This is what many people do, and it is valid. But perhaps there are also ways of progressing *within* an asana. If so, you could go on practicing Yoga creatively even if your repertoire of asanas were limited—either because you had the opportunity to learn only a few, or because your body will not permit you to advance much beyond the basic ones.

As an example let us consider Arc (*Shalabhasana*), several versions of which were included in Chapter 5.[5] The easiest way to approach this pose is to do a somewhat simplified version. Swimmer (literally, "Half" Shalabhasana), is one such. Here it is necessary only to lift one leg and one arm:

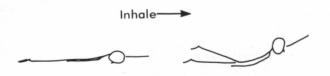

Having first practiced dynamically, you can stay for one or more breaths each way.

When you are adept at Swimmer you can start to practice Arc as well. Naturally, you would begin with a relatively easy variation, like the following:

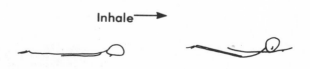

Inhaling, lift the legs while at the same time lifting and extending the arms sideward. Exhaling, return legs, chest, and arms to the mat. When you can repeat comfortably several times, you might try staying in the pose for several breaths.

Keeping to the same order—dynamic first, static after—you can try progressively more difficult variations. For example, you may sweep the arms all the way forward until the hands come together:

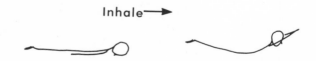

Or you may begin from Cobra and keep the chest and arms raised throughout, while lifting the legs on inhalation (as in Chapter 5, Version 2):

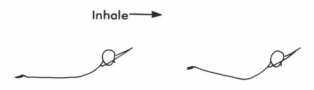

Or you may keep the palms pressed together, even on exhalation (as in Version 3):

Exhale ⟶

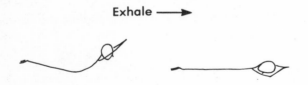

Or you may keep the *legs* raised throughout, lowering the chest and arms on exhalation:

Exhale ⟶

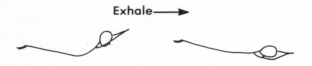

You are, of course, free to do two or more of these variations in sequence, spending several breaths on each. Eventually, you will progress to the point where you can remain in the final pose for a number of breaths:

But even then you are not through. You can now begin to use the breath to deepen the effect of the pose. First, see for how many breaths you can comfortably stay in Arc. Then see whether you can increase those breaths. One way is through retention, as described in the previous chapter, in the context of pranayama. Inhale and hold the breath for a few seconds before exhaling. (In asanas where exhalation is more easily controlled, you can also practice holding *after* exhaling—i.e., suspension).

Attention to the breath can liven up any asana. It is not necessary to keep increasing the number of repetitions in order to maintain a slight overload; instead, you can stay in the pose for progressively

more and longer breaths. If you can do Arc 6 times dynamically, see if you can do it 4 times, pausing for a breath after each elevation. Next time, see if you can increase to 6 repetitions, but remaining for a breath each time. This is one way to progress. Subsequently you can try staying in the pose for more than one breath. You might, for example, compare the effect of staying 2 breaths 3 times with staying 3 breaths 2 times.

There is no reason for asanas to become boring. Rather, the more comfortable you are in an asana, the more leeway you have for improvisation. In the case of Arc, there are still many more ways you could improvise. You could try spreading the legs on inhalation (as in Version 1) and observe the effect:

Inhale ⟶

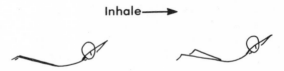

Or you could experiment with other arm positions, such as locking the hands behind the back:

Inhale ⟶

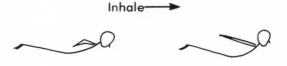

Holding a book between the knees or the palms will greatly intensify the effect:

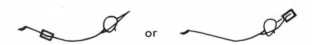

or

Or you could couple Arc with an asana having a largely opposite effect, such as Sitting Stretch:

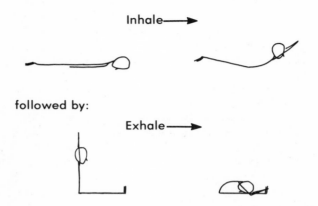

Inhale⟶

followed by:

Exhale⟶

Arc may feel different when immediately pre-ceded by Sitting Stretch. You can thus improvise, not only within an asana, but by juxtaposing one asana with another.

Improvisation in asana is limited only by your imagination, your intent, and, of course, your physical condition. No basic asana need ever be abandoned; if you outgrow one variation you can devise others to serve you better. Among the varia-tions of Arc suggested above are some you may never quite master.

This is not to say you must exhaust all possibili-ties in an asana before attempting another one of the same genre. While still working with Arc, you can in the meantime begin practicing Bow (*Dhanur-āsana*) for example, though, in its final form, it may be more advanced than Arc:

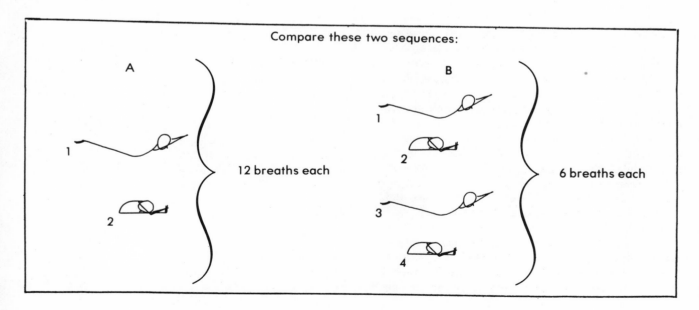

119

The point is, simply, that you need feel no compulsion to be doing new asanas as long as old ones can be made interesting. Asanas exist not to be mastered and discarded, but to be continually available as vehicles for discovery and progress.

We can sum up and generalize the stages by which we can progress within an asana as follows:

1. Asana simplified: dynamic.
2. Asana simplified: static.
3. More advanced variations: dynamic.
4. More advanced variations: static.
5. Final pose: static.
6. Increasing attention to breath (prolonging and holding).
7. Improvisation (possible at every stage).

AN OBJECTIVE

Like any other activity, Yoga is most rewarding when it is done with some object or motive. Practicing in a casual, aimless way may be pleasant enough, but it is inefficient and unfocused. When you practice without a purpose, you are less likely to improve and to recognize areas where improvement is needed. Of course any objective is only tentative. As we have seen, one function of the prelude is to allow a last-minute alteration or refinement of the objective, in keeping with the actual condition of the body.

One of the classic objectives of a Yoga course is to spend some time in Headstand. The decision to do so has a great bearing on the remainder of the course, since no other basic asana requires such careful preparation and compensation. Or your objective may be to concentrate on Shoulderstand, whether or not you decide to do Headstand as well.

OUTLINE FOR A BASIC COURSE

Planning your course around Headstand/Shoulderstand or Shoulderstand alone, you would be working within the following basic pattern:

1. Prelude: standing or otherwise.
2. Supine: preparation for inversion.
3. Inversion: (Headstand and) Shoulderstand.
4. Backbending: prone or otherwise.
5. Sitting or supine stretches.
6. Pranayama.

It goes without saying that you can rest after each of these groups—particularly before pranayama. Schematically, the sequence looks like this:

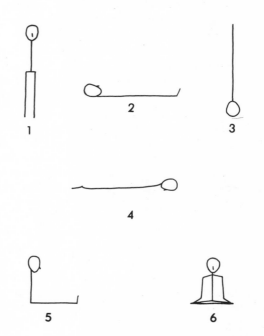

120

A course for general fitness should include a variety of trunk movements—flexion, extension, rotation—in a variety of postures—standing, sitting, lying, and inverted. It should be designed to develop strength as well as flexibility. If you are strong but stiff, you should include dynamic movements in postures that are not too awkward for you. If you are supple but weak, you should try to stay longer in basic postures. These are extremes, of course. Most people are supple in some areas and stiff in others. Try always to work toward a balance between suppleness and strength. And whether you are working dynamically or statically, make sure that you are breathing consciously and correctly.

OTHER OBJECTIVES

If you have difficulty with Headstand, one of your objectives could be to pave the way for it by practicing asanas which develop the necessary strength and poise.[6] If even Shoulderstand is hard for you, then you need to concentrate on still more basic asanas. This can be your objective for the time being.

If you don't feel like doing inverted postures you have more freedom to rearrange the items, and time to include more asanas. So long as you begin with a prelude, rest at the end, and are scrupulous about preparing and compensating for the more demanding asanas, the actual order of events is up to you.

It is a good idea to have an objective for each practice, though it may be no more than the desire to work toward a particular asana about which you have been thinking. Of course, the objective should always reflect your present state of body and mind. Don't plan a lengthy course if you have only a short time to practice, nor a strenuous course if you are feeling run-down.

As we have hinted in several places, Yoga may be of significant therapeutic value. Unfortunately, no book can do more than hint at such possibilities; prescription is impossible since individuals and conditions are always unique. Any statements we might formulate about using asanas and breathing to treat specific problems would be so riddled with contingencies as to be useless. Yoga has enormous potential when it comes to helping individuals, but cannot be implemented except by a skilled teacher, ideally in a one-to-one situation. Group classes and impersonal teaching media (including this book) simply cannot do justice to the subtler dimensions of Yoga practice.

Though we cannot deal here with specific problems you may have, it is no less true that these must be reflected in the composition of your Yoga course. Naturally they will take precedence over any other objectives you might arbitrarily set for yourself. The course objectives we have discussed so far apply only to a hypothetical person with no pressing problems; they may not apply to you. Perhaps you suffer from high blood pressure, a heart condition, some physical disability or injury, a bad back or neck, arthritis, sexual dysfunction, diabetes, obesity, ulcers or other digestive ailments, constipation, hemorrhoids, insomnia, migraines, visual problems, asthma or other respiratory problems, cancer in some form.... If so, your objective will naturally be to reduce your suffering in whatever ways you can. Yoga may be of great help in relieving pain and (at least in some cases) alleviating the problem itself. Needless to say, you will need a good teacher and lots of patience. Exactly which asanas you should practice and how you should design your course, no book can tell you, but hopefully we have given you some idea as to the direction you might proceed in.

In composing your own course, yet another legitimate objective is simply to prepare physically for a good session of pranayama. This would involve, in general, the usual prelude, followed by a group of asanas (on the back, lying face down, kneeling, sitting) to limber up the hips and back for extended sitting. Using asanas to deepen your breathing is efficient: it allows you to make the most of the time during which you can comfortably sit for the sole purpose of breathing. Headstand and Shoulderstand do help to deepen the breath, but they will make the course longer. You need not include them if you have limited time and are mainly interested in a leisurely pranayama.

PLANNING YOUR PRANAYAMA

Your final decisions in planning a course have to do with pranayama:

- Shall I include it at all?
- How long shall I spend on it?
- What sort of ratio shall I use?
- What absolute values?
- Which technique will be most appropriate?

Answers to the first two questions depend on how you feel and how much time you have. Selecting a *ratio* depends on your purpose. If you want a relaxing pranayama, make the exhalations long, relative to the inhalations. The classic proportion is 1:2, though you may add a small amount of holding. For a more vigorous pranayama, you can lengthen the inhalation so that it is equal to exhalation (1:1). You can also build toward significant retention, suspension, or both.

The *absolute values* you insert into these ratios depend on the length of your breath cycle. This is easily determined seated on a chair, after you have warmed up using asanas. Count how many seconds elapse between the start of an inhalation and the start of the next inhalation. Do this several times,

without forcing the breath, to obtain an average figure. When you come to pranayama, take this figure, reduce it sightly (just to be safe), and contrive the ratio so that the total of inhalation and exhalation does not exceed it. This is your starting pranayama; you can then increase it progressively.

For example, let us say your total breath span in asana is 14 seconds. Choose a ratio for pranayama so that inhalation and exhalation add up to no more than 14 seconds. You might aim for 12. If you want to do 1:2, start with 4.0.8.0 (i.e., 4 seconds inhalation, 8 seconds exhalation). This can be extended later by means of holding: 4.4.8.0, 4.4.8.4, etc. If you prefer to breathe in the ratio 1:1, try 6.0.6.0. This too can be progressively extended: 6.3.6.0, 6.3.6.3, 6.6.6.0, etc.

It is not imperative that you measure all of your breaths. One valid way of doing pranayama (useful also in asanas) is to count only during one or two of the phases. Examples are: inhale free (i.e., unmeasured), hold 5, exhale free; inhale free, exhale free, hold 5; inhale free, exhale 10; etc.

The *technique* you choose depends, in turn, on the ratio, the absolute values, and your purpose. Throat-sound breathing is basic, and may be used with any ratio. Single-nostril breathing (inhaling, exhaling, or both) generally permits additional control, so it is helpful where you are trying to extend one or more phases of the breath. Other varieties, such as Shitali, also have their uses.[7]

Having decided on a ratio, an appropriate technique, and feasible absolute values to start with, you can proceed to build. Just be sure you do so in easy stages. And remember that it is legitimate to interrupt your pranayama at any point for a few ordinary breaths.

We have stressed the importance of preparing for a pranayama by first breathing in an easier one: either with smaller absolute values, or using the same values but without holding the breath. (The figure "0" in a given ratio—e.g., 1:0:2:0—is of course not to be taken literally; you should always pause at least a second or two after completion of inhalation or exhalation before reversing the breath.) A well-designed course of pranayama starts easy—easy for *you*; never mind what's easy for your friend, or what a book tells you ought to be easy—builds to a sustained effort, and tapers off.

Any strenuous or concerted activity should be followed by a gradual abatement of effort. This is only common sense, and applies as much to Yoga as to athletics. Just as you warm up beforehand, you must "cool down" afterward. We saw how seated and supine postures accomplish this end within a course of asanas.

In pranayama, the passage from effort to rest has two distinct stages, though the first may be omitted if the pranayama is of the relaxing type to begin with. If it isn't—if it involves long inhalations, retention, suspension, or an extended time span even in an otherwise relaxing ratio—you should not stop abruptly, but rather scale down to normal breathing through several cycles of modest breaths in a basic ratio. For example, if your principal pranayama was 6.6.12, do at least half as many breaths of 6.0.12 before stopping. If your pranayama was 8.8.8, first drop back to 8.0.8.

Here are some hypothetical courses:

a)

5. 5.10	
5. 5.10	
5.10.10	6 breaths each
5. 0.10	

b)

8. 0.8	
8. 4.8	
8. 8.8	4 breaths each
8.12.8	
8. 0.8	

c)

10.0.10.0	
10.5.10.0	
10.5.10.5	6 breaths each
10.0.10.0	

d)

Inhale free, exhale 10   —16 breaths

e)

Inhale free, hold 4, exhale free	
Inhale free, hold 8, exhale free	8 breaths each
Inhale free, hold 0, exhale free	

As the examples suggest, a total of 16-24 breaths may be a reasonable minimum for a session—but we cannot repeat too often how much your Yoga must depend on *you*: your body, your attitude, your time, your interest, the way you feel today. A course of pranayama which is comfortable and effective for you may be far too demanding for another. Then again, tomorrow it might not even feel right to you! In setting limits to a course you must be flexible.

THE PAY-OFF

In the second stage you discontinue any further attempt at conscious control and let the breath return to normal at its own pace. To be sure, "normal" will gradually take on a new meaning, since, if you have been doing pranayama properly, even your unconscious breathing will be of a higher quality. You will be more effectively using and co-ordinating your respiratory muscles, your capacity will be greater, and your rate will be both slower and steadier.

The physiological advantages of tapering off are obvious, but there are psychological dividends too—especially during this second, or resting, stage. Now you need no longer think about your breath. You have fully exercised it, as you have previously exercised your entire body. You have sown well; this is your chance to reap—and the beauty of it is, you don't have to *do* anything! Just sit. Just breathe. Just be. If thoughts come, fine; they are likely to be important ones. Don't try to repress them. You may get some good ideas, or feel more certain about decisions recently or yet to be taken. If no thoughts of consequence arise, that's also fine; maybe you've been thinking too much lately and needed to clear your head. Don't fret. Don't struggle.

If you practice some form of meditation, this is the ideal time to do it. If not, you may get the same benefits simply by sitting. If you do your Yoga in the morning, this is the moment to tune in to your energy and vitality, to make plans, to feel the freshness of the day. If yours is an evening practice, what better time to reconsider the events of the day, your reactions and interactions? Actually, you needn't even make the effort; recollections and insights will well up unbidden—if you let them!

Put a little unstructured sitting into your life. Don't be in a hurry to get up. Having invested so much precious time in your Yoga practice, don't deny yourself the reward that comes after asana and pranayama.

A WORD TO THE WISE

However intelligently you plan your course, there is always a chance that something may go wrong. Though the body is truly an amazing machine, it is unpredictable. Even a well-designed Yoga course can backfire if you practice it blindly. So, after all our enthusiasm about the practice of asana and pranayama, we must end with a word of caution; namely, *Observe!* Accurate observation requires experience and intuition, but an attitude of observing can surely be practiced.

You will usually know whether Yoga is doing good things for you, but be on the lookout for negative evidence. There are four simple signals of overexertion in Yoga. Discontinue the exercise and rest:

1. If you feel discomfort.
2. If your mind persists in straying.
3. If there is trembling anywhere in the body.
4. If your breath becomes short.

Any one of these is sufficient cause. The fact that you pay scant attention to what you are doing in activities far more hazardous than Yoga is no reason to be reckless in Yoga as well. Let there be at least one small part of your life which is immune to expediency and coercion. If you can keep your Yoga qualitatively different from the rest of your life, perhaps the rest of your life will begin to mirror your Yoga.

REFERENCES AND NOTES

Chapter 1

[1] Loren Eiseley, The *Invisible Pyramid* (New York: Charles Scribner's Sons, 1970), pp. 146-47.

[2] William H. McNeill, *Plagues and Peoples* (Garden City, New York: Anchor Press/Doubleday, 1976), pp. 92-93.

[3] *Ibid.*, p. 94.

[4] See, for example, the chapter on "Buddhist Economics" in E. F. Schumacher, *Small is Beautiful* (London: Blond and Briggs, 1973; New York: Harper & Row, 1975).

[5] Franklin Edgerton, *The Beginnings of Indian Philosophy (London: George Allen & Unwin Ltd., 1965), p. 37 (text and footnote).*

[6] *Ibid.*, p. 37.

[7] *Ibid.*, p. 39.

[8] Henry David Thoreau, *Walden* (published in 1854), "Solitude."

[9] New York: Harper's Magazine Press, 1974.

[10] New York: William Morrow and Co., Inc., 1974.

[11] H. Chandler Elliott, *The Shape of Intelligence: The Evolution of the Human Brain* (New York: Charles Scribner's Sons, 1969), p. 279.

[12] Vaughan Thomas, *Exercise Physiology* (London: Crosby Lockwood Staples, 1975), pp. 36-37.

Chapter 6

[1] Steven F. Brena, M.D., *Yoga & Medicine* Baltimore: Penguin Books Inc, 1972), p. 84.

[2] *Breakfast of Champions* (New York: Delacorte Press/Seymour Lawrence, 1973), pp. 288-89.

[3] H. Chandler Elliott, *The Shape of Intelligence: The Evolution of the Human Brain* (New York: Charles Scribner's Sons, 1969), p. 75.

[4] *Ibid.*, p. 74.

[5] Herbert Benson, M.D., with Miriam Z. Klipper, *The Relaxation Response* (New York: William Morrow and Co., Inc., 1975; Avon Books, 1976).

[6] Brena, *Yoga & Medicine,* p. 83.

Chapter 7

[1] Lecture given on May 8, 1976; published by Cambridge Yoga Publications, 5 Long Road, Comberton, Cambridge, England. Quoted by permission.

Chapter 9

[1] Refer back to page 38.

[2] See pages 35-35.

[3] See pages 38-40 and 97.

[4] See pages 33 and 83.

[5] See pages 67-68.

[6] Such as those listed on Chapter 7 as "prerequisites" (pages 95-96).

[7] Refer back to Chapter 8, "Varieties of Pranayama" (pages 104-109).

QUEST BOOKS

are published by
The Theosophical Society in America,
a branch of a world organization
dedicated to the promotion of brotherhood and
the encouragement of the study of religion,
philosophy, and science, to the end that man may
better understand himself and his place in
the universe. The Society stands for complete
freedom of individual search and belief.
In the Theosophical Classics Series
well-known occult works are made
available in popular editions.

We have more books on yoga and on such subjects as astrology, healing, health and diet, occultism, ESP, mysticism, philosophy, psychology, religion, theosophy, and meditation. Write to us for our complete catalog.

QUEST BOOKS
306 West Geneva Road
Wheaton, Illinois 60187